Wellness
AT
Work

Building Resilience to Job Stress

Valerie O'Hara, Ph.D.

NEW HARBINGER PUBLICATIONS, INC.

Copyright © 1995 Valerie O'Hara
        New Harbinger Publications, Inc.
        5674 Shattuck Avenue
        Oakland, CA 94609

Cover design by Pamela Biery.
Text design by Tracy Marie Powell.

Distributed in U.S.A. primarily by Publishers Group West; in Canada by Raincoast Books; in Great Britain by Airlift Book Company, Ltd.; in South Africa by Real Books, Ltd.; in Australia by Boobook; in New Zealand by Tandem Press.

Library of Congress Catalog Card Number: 95-69482

ISBN 1-57224-031-8 hardcover
ISBN 1-57224-030-X paperback

Printed in Canada on recycled paper.

First printing 1995, 5,000 copies

To Ammachi for your inspiration and example.

To Ridge, Rob and Gale for your constant support, encouragement, and love.

What Is Success?

To laugh often and much;

To win the respect of intelligent people
and the affection of children;

To earn the appreciation of honest critics and
endure the betrayal of false friends;

To appreciate beauty;

To find the best in others;

To leave the world a bit better, whether by
a healthy child, a garden
patch or a redeemed social condition;

To know even one life has breathed
easier because you have lived;

This is to have succeeded.

—Ralph Waldo Emerson

Contents

Part II: Elements of a Wellness Program

Part III: Professional Services

Part IV: For Managers and Employers

About the Author

Wellness at Work is truly the result of my own life experience. I was blessed with physical and mental health and was encouraged to explore sports, personal growth, and spirituality from an early age. When I was seven years old, my mother contracted multiple sclerosis. The stress of her illness for herself and our family system opened the floodgates to my lifelong search for the meaning of life, and my investigation of the field of health and healing.

As much for our mother as for ourselves, all four children became very active physically. I greatly enjoyed ice skating, dance, and gymnastics. After attaining the United States Figure Skating Association's ranking of Gold Medalist at 18 (similar to the top degree black belt in judo or a Ph.D. in academics), and performing in an ice show, I became an international ice skating coach.

To expand my knowledge of movement, I studied yoga, and then investigated its more subtle aspects of breathing techniques and meditation. It had such an impact on my health and well-being that I decided to become a yoga teacher. After teaching yoga for 12 years, I pursued my interest in health and healing by getting a Ph.D. in psychology and becoming a stress management consultant and Marriage Family Child Counselor.

I came to see how important self-knowledge and self-care are for vibrant health and happiness. I gradually realized all the avenues I had been exploring combined into an integrated wellness approach to life. I recognized how effective the tools I had learned could be for people who are experiencing stress. In 1988 I founded the La Jolla Institute for Stress Management and created The Fitness Option Program, which became the basis for my first book, *The Fitness Option*. I taught many of its concepts at the University of California at San Diego. The students very sweetly dubbed their class time with me as "an oasis."

Since writing *The Fitness Option*, more and more clients have come in seeking counseling due to job stress. This motivated me to examine statistics on anxiety, depression, job burnout, personality types prone to job stress, and ways to alleviate job stress. *Wellness at Work* is my antidote to your job stress: a personalized Wellness Program coupled with suggestions for restructuring the workplace to make it caring and personally sensitive, while remaining efficient and profitable.

This book is to aid you, the reader, in overcoming job stress. May reading *Wellness at Work* lead to expanded horizons and an increased sense of well-being and happiness.

Acknowledgments

This morning my first words were, "I'm excited and happy. I get to work on my book today." From its inception, the writing of this book has been a very positive experience for me. I wrote on weekends and one day during the week while continuing my counseling practice, and it turned out to be a wonderful balance to the other parts of my life. My enthusiasm in sharing this material is a reflection of my long-term success in using the techniques for stress management in my own life and in counseling my clients. The acknowledgments therefore will not include thanking my husband for putting up with my irritability! On the contrary, he is looking forward to my next book project!

Writing a book is not something I would want to do alone. It would be lonely and boring and the end product less than what it could be. This project has been a joint enterprise from the beginning. I have appreciated connecting with strangers, friends, and colleagues. Each phase, from research, to writing, to editing and design has brought new or deepened relationships into my life. I have enjoyed the richness of the project. I hope you, the reader, receive great benefit from the effort of many.

Special thanks goes to those numerous kind people I met on the telephone, especially those in government document offices, who took their time to lead me through the bureaucratic maze to uncover up-to-date statistics. I never saw the inside of a library! Almost daily, for the first four months of writing, the raw data poured in. I was like a teenager in love, as I expectantly waited for the mail each day!

Special gratitude to my two editors, Gail Perryman and Rob Whittemore. I appreciated Gail's diligent efforts to keep the book user-friendly by suggesting more case histories, examples, and reader-participation exercises. I valued and followed her perceptive suggestions. My brother Rob, in his typical fashion, jumped in with both feet when I asked him to read the manuscript. He went way beyond a cursory reading. After entering the manuscript into his computer, we faxed and talked on the telephone for months as he honed in on details, seeking clarification and validation for the sake of the reader. I thank Matt McKay, my publisher, for his faith in me and his enthusiasm for the project. Heartfelt thanks to Allen Schmeltz for his excellent photography of the office exercises.

I acknowledge my clients as a source of inspiration. They overcame monumental stress with determination, perseverance, and willingness to change. I learned from each of them.

I thank my husband, Bryan, who was a constant support for me throughout the whole process, with his enthusiastic energy and practical, professional comments. Our discussions became a special sharing time for us. Without him there would be no book!

How To Use *Wellness at Work*

You are successful the moment you start moving toward a worthwhile goal.

—Caption for "Success," a photograph by
Charles Carlson (The Executive Gallery)

Wellness at Work gives you a structure for managing job stress—to make definitive changes that will restore your enthusiasm, increase your productivity, and give you peace of mind at work. It helps you pinpoint what is stressing you. It helps you understand exactly how the stressors affect you—physically, mentally, and emotionally. It offers specific techniques to reduce both the symptoms and the causes of your current stress as well as to build your resiliency to future stress. It provides exercises for you to apply these techniques at work and to develop your own wellness program.

First, learn what is going on with you. Part I describes the physiological and mental aspects of stress and presents a checklist of work site stressors for you to determine the relevant factors in your job that are disturbing you. This is followed by a series of checklists to help you pinpoint precisely how you react to the stressors of your job. These checklists measure your physical, emotional, and behavioral responses to stress including assessing for anxiety and depression, examining your personality type for vulnerability to stress, and determining your degree of job burnout. At the end of Part I, you will combine the results of these checklists to create your personal Stress Profile.

Second, retrain your mind and body to habits of wellness. Part II presents hands-on techniques to relieve your stress symptoms. These techniques include relaxation training, aerobic activities, office exercises, cognitive remedies, nutritional tools, tools to improve communication, and suggestions for expanding your social support and self-care activities. By practicing each technique as you work through the book, you will discover which techniques are most effective for you. At the end of Part II, you will combine your favorite applications to create your personal Wellness Program.

Third, learn what professional services are available to you. Part III outlines professional options that are available when you are feeling so overwhelmed by stress that you are unable to set your own self-help strategies into motion.

Fourth, discover what management can do to ease employee stress. Part IV advises managers on the benefits of employee wellness and offers suggestions, including how to increase employee self-esteem. It discusses the financial advantages of instituting mental health programs and fitness classes for employees.

Throughout the book, I provide case examples from my counseling practice to bring alive clinical descriptions of stress patterns, and for you to discover that you are not alone. To protect the identity of my clients, I have changed all the names, locations, and corporate titles, and created composite characters. Although fictitious, they are not exaggerated, and represent the norm experienced in job stress.

Introduction

Creating a better future starts with the ability to envision it.

—Caption for "Vision," a photograph
(The Executive Gallery)

What a precious gift life is! Each day we choose how to live this priceless treasure. When we are at peace and harmony with ourselves and others, we perceive its beauty, joy, and challenge. When life is seen as exciting and filled with opportunity, stress is the spice of life. It motivates us to achieve more, to be enthusiastic, happy, and full of energy. When we doubt ourselves, distrust those around us, or are overwhelmed by too much input, the gift becomes tarnished; the dream becomes a nightmare. A spicy stimulus becomes poison if we are overcome by it (Brailler, 1982). Stress as a stimulator becomes dis-ease and dis-comfort when it negatively affects our body, mind, or spirit.

We understand better than ever before the physiology of stress, the effect of stress on the emotions, and the role of the mind in creating stress. This knowledge has resulted in better solutions to the detrimental effects of stress.

Ironically, stress is not only better understood but also more pervasive than ever before. The pressures of life have always been with us; our fears of the unknown and our struggles to survive are as old as history itself. But stress as we now understand and experience it has new facets. It is a household and job site word and synonymous with the modern age.

Our highly technological society and demanding life styles have aggravated and exacerbated the negative impact of stress. In past eras from the Stone Age to Medieval times man knew less about the world around him but faced life as part of a community. The extended family and support system of fellow tribesmen gave a sense of security and kinship that helped to ease the struggles of life. As we have modernized and technologized, we have also individualized. We now live in immediate family units, commute individually or with indifferent strangers, and work at specialized stations or at home, alone. The traditional support systems have broken down and are only partially replaced by support groups, church, or community activities.

Technological inventions such as satellite dishes and cable television have brought the world into our living rooms. When we are personally unable to cope with our own lives, news scenes of city violence and crime, footage of war in foreign countries, newspaper reports of natural and ecological disasters add to our sense of overwhelm.

Technology has also allowed us to become more sedentary at home and at work. Many people sit all day at a computer terminal or assembly line and then sit through the evening watching television. Daily pressures—emotional fervor and physical tension—are not being naturally discharged or released through physical activity. This chronic buildup of stress results in physical and emotional imbalance.

The shrinkage of time and space through cellular phones, fax machines, and laser printers demands speeded up responses and a steeper learning curve to assimilate the information flood. Work environments with no windows, artificial lighting, few living plants, uncomfortable work stations, or a high level of noise pollution add to job dissatisfaction. The efficiency, comfort, and convenience created by modern technology has simultaneously introduced new challenges to managing stress.

My Personal Experience with Job Stress

My own story illustrates the painful impact of stress. Five years ago I started experiencing disturbed sleep patterns. At 4 a.m. my mind began to churn; I tossed and turned as ideas and plans bounced through the labyrinth of my mind. During the day, my natural enthusiasm ebbed to a mere trickle of energy. I became fatigued, irritable, and on the verge of tears. Looking back now, it seems clear that my decline began with enthusiastic involvement in more and more projects. I was wearing the various hats of counselor, director, and teacher. In the wee hours of the morning, I was the mail order distributor of my book, video, and audiotapes. Over a period of a year, I had done what so many of us do. To gain time, I stopped exercising, cut out any social life, ceased doing yoga postures and meditation, and ignored both physical and emotional responses to overload. I continued to press on, doing essentially three jobs at once. After directing and teaching a full-time Wellness Program during the day, I would jump in my car and race 25 minutes to meet my first counseling appointment at 4:30 p.m. Late in the evening I would return home to the mail orders from my book, video, and audiotapes on stress management! I'd sort the mail, wrap packages, apply labels and tape, and write out the UPS and Federal Express forms. After dragging myself to bed, I'd be annoyed that I couldn't get to sleep. I'd set the alarm to wake myself as early as possible to prepare for my morning classes on, ironically, how to overcome stress!

Finally, I experienced panic attacks. These attacks were a frightening signal for me to pay attention to symptoms of excess stress. Fortunately, I recognized what I was doing to myself, and took action. One month after reinstating the healthy habits I had dropped, the panic attacks and migraines stopped. After eight months my blood pressure was sufficiently low enough to satisfy my doctor that I did not need medication. My enthusiasm and energy returned when I set realistic goals and gave myself permission to relax, to be creative, and to enjoy the small pleasures in life such as drinking a cup of tea with a friend, or taking a walk in the woods. I made work changes, too, delegating some jobs and focusing on other jobs with fuller attention.

I learned my lesson well, and the result is the book you hold in your hands.

My encounter with job stress is part of an epidemic. In the United States, over 75 percent of all visits to primary care physicians are to treat stress-related complaints, and the vast majority of these complaints are job-related (Wallace, 1992). Work site stress can kill the very spirit of who we are as individuals. Our dreams, aspirations, creative goals, and hopes to "make a difference" wither and die if the stress of daily work obscures our capabilities.

The Solution: Taking Charge of Your Wellness

Too often people do not recognize the symptoms of stress or do not realize they can do something about their pain. You can do so much to feel better about yourself and your job situation. It is gratifying to know that you can take charge of your life and personally improve your health and well-being—and avoid the high costs of health care and the draining effects of stress. Committing yourself to a Wellness Program consisting of regular exercise, relaxation time, and good nutrition, coupled with improved communication skills, positive perceptions, and enhanced self-esteem will reduce your job stress to a manageable level.

Don't wait! When you are feeling down or anxious, when you are having trouble sleeping, when you are feeling stressed, take action as soon as you can to take care of yourself. Like flashing red lights, these are signals from your body, mind, and spirit that you are out of balance. Don't disregard your warning signs.

Creating wellness at work needs to be both an individual and collective act. *Wellness at Work* offers solutions to job stress for both employees and managers. Business managers, I believe, have a duty: they are responsible as stewards of the workplace for providing a wholesome environment for their employees, and the simple fact is that happy, healthy workers create better products and more profits.

Expanding the awareness and coping skills of employees and restructuring and humanizing the corporate structure will overpower the strangulating grip of stress.

I feel good when I take care of myself and when I appreciate the gift of life and health I have been given. Many of us suffer, not from the trials and challenges of the job, but from our lack of self-worth and self-care. These are challenges we can meet.

You too can manage stress and have wellness. The harmful effects of workplace stress can be eradicated. You can become a victorious warrior in the battle of life rather than a victim. Make the decision to take command of your life. You can do what is necessary to conquer stress.

Part I

UNDERSTANDING AND MEASURING WORKPLACE STRESS

1

Dynamic Wellness

There are seven sections to cross on the bridge to Wellness: a quiet mind, exercise, nutrition, de-addiction, safety, lovingness, and ethical behavior.

—Dr. Edward Taub, *Prescription for Life*

Developing wellness is the first and foremost solution to job stress or difficulties of any kind. But what does that mean? What kind of wellness is so profound, and has such resilience, as to be immune to the stress epidemic? There is such wellness, and you can be that well, even at work.

Wellness at work is the active art of building resilience to job stress and daily life. It is more than the absence of illness—it is an approach to life. Wellness embraces the best of who we are in body, mind, and spirit. It is proactive and preventive. It touches every part of our life by emphasizing good health care, cultivating self-awareness, living according to our values and beliefs, being our own best friend, and realizing the value of family, friends, and coworkers. Wellness is feeling enthusiasm for life, enjoying self-discovery and growth. It is saying "Yes!" to the challenges of life.

Developing Wellness at Work

What does this kind of wellness look like and how is it related to work?

1. Wellness is attention to self-care details such as choosing shoes that fit, knowing your cholesterol level, wearing sun screen, and getting a yearly checkup. It is buckling your seat belt and flossing your teeth. It means making time, no matter what your workload, to take care of yourself.

2. Wellness is expanding your awareness of how you are feeling and perceiving yourself and life around you. It is learning how to let go of those emotions and images that are imprisoning you. It is recognizing the importance of balancing personal quiet time and creativity with work and other responsibilities. Wellness is caring enough about yourself to want to discover more about you. It emphasizes developing your potential both inside and outside of the workplace.

3. Wellness is practicing financial integrity and balance. This includes being realistic in expenditures. When we stretch the budget to meet endless desires, our comfort zone is eroded. Financial stress dissolves when we live within our means. Financial wellness includes learning to discriminate between healthy needs and endless transient desires. Work is an important part of life, but wellness is working to live, not living to work.

4. Wellness is the acceptance that we are not alone and separate, but part of a whole. Wellness is flowing with circumstances and people, not needing to dominate and control them. Just as we are beginning to reclaim and nurture the planet we have damaged, so must we extend this sense of unity and wholeness to our personal workplace.

5. For management, wellness at work is broadening the profit motive to embrace the needs and concerns of the employee as to the importance of teamwork and grass roots decision-making. It is Wellness Programs and good health benefits for the employee. It is a sense of family.

6. Wellness is growing larger in relation to the challenge we are facing. No matter what the trials of life, suffering can be minimized by growing larger in your relationship to them through increasing self-esteem. Stress, dissatisfaction, anxiety, and depression all signify a diminished sense of self-empowerment. Wellness at work means responding on the job from an inner strength, confidence, or sense of calm.

7. Wellness is the process of becoming. It is the carving away of all that you are not, to reveal your strength, harmony, joy, and wisdom. It is putting joy back into your work life and personal life.

Basic Elements of a Wellness Program

Needed: Willingness for the Journey

To embark on the Wellness Journey, begin by taking stock of who you are now. This takes a willingness to face your habits, faults, and perceptions. It takes courage to assess your physical, emotional, and spiritual selves. This first step—self-awareness—includes accepting what you discover. Only then can you embrace growth. The assessments in Part I are designed to help you identify your work-related stressors and responses.

Tend Your Body

Rarely do we appreciate the blessings of health. Think of your body as a window pane. When the glass is clean you are unaware of it as you enjoy the view beyond. If it is streaked with mud, scratched, cracked, or broken, it takes great effort to see, much less appreciate, the view. It takes tremendous energy to live with an ill or stressed body. Only when we are diseased or injured do we appreciate the blessing of a healthy body.

Stress, specifically job stress, puts wear and tear on the body and exacerbates genetic tendencies. A commitment to good health care can mitigate or even prevent physical disease due to stress. The stress management skills in Part II that include good nutrition, enjoyable exercise, regular practice of relaxation skills such as breathing techniques, muscular relaxation, yoga, and visualization, are the cornerstones of preventive medicine and wellness.

Observe Your Mind

The mind is a chatterbox. We have come to accept a stream—*a torrent*—of internal self-talk. Most of it is comparative, judgmental, or critical of oneself or others. The mind dwells on past grievances or future worries. Although preparedness is beneficial, and learning from one's mistakes is admirable, how many times does your mind repeat the same tape over and over? It's stuck on automatic replay.

When you dwell on past events or future worries, you miss out on the joy of life by not being in the present moment. Learn how to let go of obsessive, nagging mental stagnation. Part II offers guidelines and exercises to help you cultivate a calm and alert mind.

Expand Your Spirit

To live your values—to listen to your conscience—is the root system of your tree of wellness. What do you believe in? Whom do you admire, respect, or cherish? The more you live according to your ideals, the greater your peace of mind and enjoyment of life. Fulfillment of your short-term desires at the expense of your long-term goals only dampens your spirit. Loyalty to your ideals, however, must be delicately balanced with accepting your shortcomings—learning from your mistakes and not berating yourself. Part II offers suggestions on how to increase self-esteem and minimize negative, limiting emotions and perceptions. It includes ways to expand your spirit through creative expression and nurturing support systems.

Conclusion

The Wellness Journey offers you the opportunity to shape your life according to your own map of inner potential. The workplace is filled with inevitable challenges that demand personal growth. The ports of call on this journey, as Dr. Edward Taub, author and nationwide lecturer on stress management and wellness, so clearly identifies, are a quiet mind, exercise, nutrition, de-addiction, safety, lovingness, and ethical behavior. The destination is enthusiasm, well-being, and a sense of peace. Begin your journey now.

2

Stress: The Disease Whose Cure Can Change Your Life

Without work, all life goes rotten, but when work is soulless, life stifles and dies.

—Albert Camus

The workplace can be an environment not only for profit, but also for companionship and laughter, for self-fulfillment and growth. It can be a source of personal satisfaction and achievement. Practicing effective antidotes to job stress can eradicate road blocks in your life's journey of self-discovery and healing.

> *Jennifer, a middle management supervisor, walked briskly into my office and sat down with a smile. "I'm on track again. I'm taking my dog, Tyler, for a walk and eating breakfast before leaving for the office. I've been relaxing with five-minute visualization breaks at work. By setting boundaries with my coworkers, I no longer feel like diving under my desk when they approach. I don't dread Mondays. I've beaten depression!"*

Do you, like Jennifer, experience stress at your job in the form of mental distraction, chronic fatigue, depression, unrelenting anxiety, nervousness, feelings of ineptitude, or a sense of being stuck in high gear? Do you cause problems for yourself or others because you have no healthy means to relieve pent-up pressures? If so, you are not alone. In fact,

75 percent of Americans surveyed described their job as stressful and feel that job pressure is steadily growing (International Labor Office, 1993).

Stress plagues our society. It has reached epidemic proportions. Its tentacles reach everywhere, unraveling the fabric of our lives. Stress is the number one disease of the modern workplace, affecting employees and employers alike; its mental, physical, and financial costs stagger the imagination.

Stress is a crisis, not an inevitable fixture in the workplace. Significantly, the character for "crisis" in the Chinese language is a composite of two characters: one denoting "danger," and the other denoting "opportunity." Will you use the warning signals of stress as the opportunity to create new, healthy options? The choice is yours.

Recognize and Respond to Early Stress Warning Signals

An important aspect of effective stress management is calling for help or making necessary changes before you are in dire straits. I learned this important lesson not only from my clients but also from my own mistake of ignoring the signs of stress presented by my body, mind, emotions, and behavior. Consider what happened to David when he disregarded his warning system.

> *David worked for a nationwide trucking firm as a maintenance supervisor. Because he did not want to upset the lives of family members, he did not move when his company reassigned him to a new location. Instead, he commuted three hours each way to and from work. This commute added to the pressures of an already exacting ten-hour-a-day job. Sometimes he slept in a motel or at a friend's home. Other times he camped out in his pickup truck and used public rest room facilities. David became ragged and edgy from lack of proper sleep. On the weekends his wife was disappointed and frustrated because all he wanted to do was rest. He couldn't relate to her life or concentrate on her problems. He was as worn out, lifeless, and limp as his faded sweat shirt. One morning he woke up in a fetal position, crying like a baby. He could do no more. It took psychiatric care, medication, months of quiet time, and quitting his job before he fully recovered.*

Too often I meet clients who have not heeded the warning signals. Recovery is more difficult if the early telltale signs of distress are ignored. Many of us, like David, think we can be heroes, do the impossible, and overlook the early stress warning signs. Don't allow this to happen to you. When job pressures first emerge as irritability, depression, insomnia, ill health, or a host of other early stress warning signs, you are stressed. Take immediate action. Observe how Paul paid attention to his physical symptoms and handled his stress crisis.

> *Paul appeared in my office slightly annoyed and restless. He is a 45-year-old handsome and muscularly built athletic coach. He is also the assistant dean of a large local high school. With*

a clenched jaw, and with rapid, clipped sentences, he declared, "I don't get it. I eat a low fat and high fiber diet with lots of organic fruits and vegetables. I work out four times a week with weights and do cardiovascular exercises. I have a full schedule of civic and school responsibilities. My classes are the largest of any teacher. My teams are winners. I do everything the books say. Can't the dean appreciate that I work twelve hour days? Can't he lay off all the extra 'little' assignments? I can't even get a break at home with my wife and all her lists of things for me to do. Now the doctor says I have ulcers, high blood pressure, and colitis. Things are looking decidedly bleak with all the doctor bills. How can I manage these costs and still save for the kids' going to college? As it is, I've become a stranger to them. Look at me! I look fine, but I'm a total wreck. What can I do?"

Paul was suffering from job stress exacerbated by "Type A" personality traits. For Paul, the extraordinary demands of essentially two jobs rolled into one (assistant dean and athletic coach), coupled with internal perfectionist pressures of being "the best," resulted in physical problems and costly medical bills. Paul found relief through counseling. We focused on his need to prioritize his duties at work and home, and how to make time for the active family life he so desired. He participated in his school's new Stress Management Program. Paul especially benefited from the program's discussion on the drawbacks of perfectionism—particularly that of setting impossible expectations for oneself and then feeling guilty for not meeting them. In the self-assessment section of this book, you will be able to examine your own "Type A" tendencies.

Costs of Stress to Society

Paul was significantly helped by his employer's Stress Management Program—part of a growing, enlightened response to the stress epidemic. Stress is now acknowledged to be one of the most serious health issues of the 20th century. Stress-related diseases not only impair individuals, but also severely impact employers and governments as well. In the United States alone, the annual cost of job-related stress is approximately $200 billion–often cloaked in the form of increased absenteeism, reduced productivity, staff turnover, accidents, compensation claims, high health insurance costs, and medical expenses (International Labor Office, 1993).

A major factor in absenteeism is poor health, particularly poor psychological well-being. In 1984 an average of one million workers were absent on any given workday, largely due to stress-related disorders. Employees who drink alcohol and smoke took twice as much time off (International Labor Office, 1993).

More than one third of America's work force finds it increasingly difficult to balance work and family life, and to cope with pressures on the job. Responses to a survey of 600 full-time employees showed:

46% felt "highly stressed."

25% believed they were suffering from stress-related illness.

69% experienced high stress and reduced productivity.

17% blamed stress for 10+ days of absenteeism for 1990.

14% quit or changed jobs in the previous two years due to job stress.

66% blamed stress for exhaustion, anger, anxiety, or muscular pain.

72% experienced three or more stress-related illnesses somewhat or very often (Walker, 1991).

In 1985 approximately 11 million workers reported "health endangering" levels of mental stress at the job site (Sauter et al., 1990). These sobering statistics are a striking indicator of the magnitude of stress in the workplace.

The Remarkably Low Cost of Recovery

Cases from my counseling practice reveal that the cost of stress is very high, and the cure is remarkably inexpensive. Let's look at an example of a modern businessman. Professional businesspeople like Ryan are modern day gunfighters, dodging the fast moving bullets of computer information and deadlines, and shooting back memos, faxes, and instant analyses. Swamped with too much knowledge to absorb and too little time for reflection or creative contemplation, they simply can't handle it all (Gibbs, 1989).

> *Ryan, CEO for a mid-sized company, dragged into my office, and slumped into a chair. Pirated one year previously from another company because of his stamina, innovative ideas, and interpersonal management skills, this serious, intelligent, and highly motivated young man was now displaying fatigue, withdrawal, and lack of enthusiasm. Three to four times weekly he awoke at 4 a.m. and could not get back to sleep due to worry about work projects and deadlines. He was overeating and not exercising. Even more alarming, he was returning to his old drinking patterns, and his wife was seriously contemplating leaving him. He was uncomfortable at staff meetings. "People are a problem," he said. "They put me down, talk behind my back, and exploit my weaknesses." He felt a sense of doom and hopelessness.*

Under the pressure of fitting into a new job and putting unrealistic demands on himself, Ryan allowed his self-esteem and healthy life style to erode. He had turned his dream of success into a living nightmare. Ryan was suffering from depression due to job stress.

Ryan instituted a multifaceted Wellness Program. He regained his self-esteem with help from counseling. He made life style changes including nutritional improvements. He instituted a walking program and practiced relaxation skills daily. On Tuesday evenings he increased his communication skills through role-playing and attending a Toast Masters program. On Wednesdays he attended the local AA meeting. On Friday and Sunday evenings he practiced a half-hour Worry Focus exercise, followed by five minutes of relaxation. After two intense months, Ryan was smiling. He declared, "I am happy and productive again."

Ryan's case demonstrates that the path to wellness at work demands a high degree of commitment to the cure, but given the severity of the illness the treatment is usually relatively inexpensive. All of the suggestions Ryan used to create his Wellness Program are in Part II. By committing yourself to regular practice of a few simple stress management skills, you, too, will find yourself feeling happier and more productive.

Even more important, the remedy for stress reaches beyond the workplace and totally transforms your life. It rejuvenates you and heads you along the path of self-discovery. Victory over stress and depression is possible if you invest willingness and effort, and hold the vision of wellness before you.

3

The Physiology of Stress

*There are pervasive anatomic and biochemical links between the
immune and nervous systems to explain the influence of mood on
susceptibility to disease.*

— J.L. Marx quoted in *Prevention of
Work-Related Psychological Disorders*

*Changing our attitudes of worry and despair to enthusiasm and
evenmindedness has a powerful healing effect.*

—Patricia Norris quoted in *Healers on Healing*

The body is often the first indicator that stress has reached the level of distress. It responds quickly to real or perceived threats. In the classic situation, if our senses tell us that our lives are in jeopardy, the body gears up for immediate battle or speed. All internal systems respond: the heart speeds up, the breath becomes more rapid, muscles tense, eyes dilate, the gastrointestinal system disrupts digestive processes, nerves and hormones respond. By this "flight or fight" stress response, we instinctively gird for action.

Extensive research in several fields of medicine and psychology, including brain chemistry, neurobiology, immunology, and psychoendocrinology, attest to the body/mind connection (Fahrion and Norris, 1990). In fact, scientifically, the body and the mind do not exist independently of each other. The limbic system known as the "emotional brain" regulates sexual impulse, pain, hunger, fear, and anger. This limbic system is the "primary responder" to psychological stress and has numerous interconnections with the hypothalamus and pituitary gland. It gathers input from our thoughts and emotions and relays the information to the hypothalamus. The hypothalamus controls the autonomic nervous system which regulates blood pressure, heartbeat, respiration, muscle tension, metabolism, and intestines. The pituitary gland, also receiving stress signals from the limbic system, releases adrenaline and other stress-related hormones (Norris and Fahrion, 1993).

Let's look at an example of how the body/mind connection handles new information. Suppose you receive a telephone call from the child care center administrator saying they will not be able to watch your child tomorrow. Your self-talk sounds something like this: "Oh, no, what am I going to do with Jane? Staying home with her is out of the question. The planning committee meets tomorrow and I could never tell my boss that I'm needed at home. Gary won't take her, Doris is away on a trip, and Mom lives 500 miles away! What am I going to do? I don't have time to deal with this today, much less tomorrow!" Now look at how your body has responded to fear thoughts: your blood pressure is up, your heart is racing, your breath is shallow, and your stomach knots—a typical stress response.

Consider another, more fanciful, example. Suppose you and the family are camping. After everyone settles in for the night, there are crashing sounds and low growling noises. You jump up shouting, "Bear!", adrenaline flowing and muscles tense. The kids break out in peals of laughter. "We fooled you!"

Consequences of Stress-Overload

The hypothalamus cannot distinguish between a real or an imagined threat. Even though the bear was imaginary, your adrenaline and muscle tension are real. Your body responds to the perceived threat the same as it would have had a bear actually lumbered into your campsite.

Your body cannot distinguish between worry thoughts and the original catastrophe. Worry thoughts act as a repeat of the threat—a false alarm. This causes the body's magnificent rapid response system to become its own undoing, because your worried mind keeps your body perpetually in high gear, muscles tense, ever ready to meet a challenge. Your body responds to repeated worrisome thoughts and emotions in essentially the same way as it responded to the original stressor. The internal emergency response system, to which we all as a species undoubtedly owe our survival, breaks down.

People who experience repeated and unrelenting stress in their lives gradually lose the ability to downshift. The wear and tear on our system shows up in the form of cardiovascular illnesses, ulcers, tension headaches, and panic attacks. Chronic irritability, impatience, depression, and frustration lead to actual tissue changes and organ malfunctions. Over-secretion of gastric acid can lead to ulcers; sustained vasoconstriction (narrowing of the blood vessels) can lead to hypertension; and colon hyperactivity can lead to spastic colon or colitis. Other common stress-related disorders include insomnia, migraine headaches, back pain, and diabetes (Pelletier, 1982).

Let's look at what can happen, physically and emotionally, when one gets stuck in a worry mode—and what can be done about it.

Stuck in Fast Forward

Carla *whisked into my office. She was edgy and restless. She is a clinical administrator at a government research laboratory, and was referred to me by her doctor. "I'm good at what I do. I've had this position for over ten years. My boss is a 'control freak,' overloads me, and sets impossible deadlines. I am only hanging on for the retirement and health benefits that I'm entitled to in four years. Every evening I sit in my favorite chair in my living room and stare into space for protracted periods, feeling overwhelmed and exhausted. I have no energy and feel depressed. I can't concentrate at home or at work. I'm always tired, but unable to sleep through the night. I have constant stomachaches and headaches. Worst of all, almost daily for the last month, 'out of the blue' my heart races, it's hard to breathe, I feel numbness and tingling in my arms, and intense chest pain. These experiences are sudden and intense but only last ten to twenty minutes. I feel like I'm going crazy. What's wrong with me?"*

Carla was not "going crazy." She was both depressed and extremely anxious. Her anxiety resulted in panic attacks—brief but intense bouts of racing heart, tightness in the chest, difficulty in breathing, and numbness. Anti-depressant and anti-anxiety medication helped Carla stabilize her condition while she learned relaxation skills and how to modify her negative, pessimistic thinking. She quit working overtime and on weekends. She no longer feels guilty when unable to meet unrealistic deadlines. She remains diligent and efficient, but honors her decision to work to live, not to live to work. She is now happy at her job and nearing retirement in good health.

Five out of six workers filing claims for illness feel that job stress is a major cause (International Labor Office, 1993). Carla's situation is unfortunately typical: performance anxiety, coupled with an organizational structure which kept her out of the decision-making process, led to illness, depression, panic attacks, and feelings of being overwhelmed and out of control.

How Stress Directly Impacts the Immune System and Health

The mind influences the immune system via the nervous system. During the mid-70s, researchers at the University of Rochester School of Medicine and Dentistry discovered this connection, and since then many experiments have shown the powerful impact of the mind on the immune system. This means that psychological distress can suppress the immune system enough to increase the risk of physical illness. According to a landmark study at Carnegie Mellon University, published in the New England Journal of Medicine, your chance of getting a cold or respiratory infection is directly proportional to the amount of stress you experience (*Consumer Reports*, 1993).

Suppressing the immune system can be far more dangerous than catching a cold. As I point out in *The Fitness Option*, the immune system—the first line of defense against infection, germs, bacteria, and toxins in our bodies—is weakened by stress. Like paramedics rushing to the scene of an accident, the immune system's neurotransmitters, lymphokines, and endorphins are first arrivals in the healing of an injury. But these powerful aids are crippled by stress messages from the brain. Fear, depression, anger, and other negative emotions depress the immune system. Bereavement, depression, loneliness, and chronic stress immobilize the natural killer cells within the immune system (O'Hara, 1990).

On the other hand, mental messages of calm or joy have been shown to be physiologically beneficial. Research at UCLA Medical Center indicates that a peaceful or happy frame of mind frequently stimulates production of interleukins, which are vital substances in the immune system that help activate cancer killing immune cells (Cousins, 1990). Fortunately, an inhibited immune system can recover if the mind's messages change from distress to calmness.

The Relaxation Response

Research on the physiology of stress shows the potency of managing stress through training yourself to elicit the mirror opposite of the flight or fight stress response: *the relaxation response*. The relaxation response reduces heart and respiration rates, blood pressure, and metabolism via the hypothalamus and generates brain rhythms associated with peace.

You can learn to elicit the relaxation response through breathing techniques, deep relaxation, guided visualization, meditation, and biofeedback. The relaxation response is a proven counterbalance to the stress response. The first section in Part II will teach you how to elicit the relaxation response at work. It is fundamental to managing stress and is a necessary element of your Wellness Program.

4

Variables in Your Resilience
to Stress

The most important product in your life is you.

—Stephen C. Paul, *Illuminations*

Everyone has a different threshold for coping with stimulation. Two primary variables affect how you meet challenges: your past experience and your personality. Understanding these two important parts of yourself will help you to cope with stressful demands in your life and work. Let's briefly explore these two factors in maintaining your wellness.

Lighting the Long Shadows of the Past

Unresolved inner tension can surface in seemingly unrelated and often inappropriate ways, and it can be particularly difficult when this happens at work. Consider what happened to Denise. She is an example of how an unresolved, painful childhood can result in a lowered threshold for handling stress.

Denise, a cashier in a major discount store, was referred to me by her supervisor to learn anger management and improve her communication skills. She was suspended because she burst out angrily when customers disagreed as to who was next in line. Pounding the counter, she had exclaimed, "I don't give a damn who's next! Sort it out yourselves." Turning on a coworker who attempted to intercede, she screamed, "Get off my back!" and stormed off to the rest room.

Chagrined by her rude behavior and anxious not to lose her job, Denise openly admitted lack of control over her temper. She acknowledged that she verbally abused her boyfriend and that she had nightmares. She also experienced chronic migraine headaches, for which she took ten aspirin daily, without much relief.

Additional therapy revealed that Denise suffered from low self-esteem and inner rage resulting from untreated childhood molestation. Through counseling, Denise mitigated her childhood rage and hurt which increased her self-esteem. This dramatically reduced her headaches and improved her ability to handle job stress. She also learned how to communicate her feelings appropriately, rather than letting them build to a rage before expressing them. This training helped her improve relationships at work and at home.

For Denise, stressful situations at work, coupled with a traumatic family history, triggered inappropriate upheavals. Once Denise no longer felt guilty or labeled herself as a "bad" person because she had been molested, she calmed down and found inner peace. Once she was more relaxed, she could begin to see current situations as disagreeable, but not necessarily a direct attack on her, and respond helpfully.

Think of your own childhood years. Did you suffer a trauma or other life crisis that has not been resolved? Present day tensions tend to awaken past unresolved pain such as depression, anger, rage, or anxiety. In this way, shadows from the past make a person more vulnerable to stress. In order to go forward in your life, strengthened rather than diminished by your experiences, past hurts need to be faced rather than buried. However, coming to terms with long-buried pain may not be something you can handle alone. You may need the support of a caring counselor or a support group. Information on finding such support is included in Part III.

Personality Types Vary in Resilience to Stress

Your personality type, which is defined by specific behaviors and emotions, affects your resilience to stress. Cardiologists Meyer Friedman and Ray Rosenman observed a correlation between specific behavior patterns and heart problems. They coined the term "Type A personality" for people with an urgent, aggressive, and hostile approach to life, and the term "Type B personality" for those who are easy-going and relaxed. Fortunately, Type A does have a positive side, and Type B personality can be cultivated.

Type A characteristics are not automatically detrimental to your health. Society even encourages some of these behaviors. Corporations seek out ambitious, hard working, and competitive individuals. Many people work long hours, fully enjoying that important part of their lives. Type A personalities largely evaluate themselves by their success at work. They may not make the best parents or spouses, and they tend to keep feelings to themselves, but this does not necessarily lead to ill health. But when these traits or habits develop into chronic dissatisfaction, anger, and hostility, a healthy Type A personality becomes an anxious, aggressive, unhappy, burned-out individual with a greatly increased risk of coronary heart disease (Klarreich, 1990).

Let's look at an example of how personality type affects one's response to job stress. Three coworkers faced an identical problem: a driving snow storm at the close of a convention. Their return flight was delayed by several hours.

> *During the delay,* **Bob** *called his wife to explain the situation, and then had a beer and watched television at the airport bar. His flexibility allowed him to easily readjust his schedule.*
>
> **Brian** *forgot to call home, but he too adjusted to the delay. He found a relatively quiet spot in the airport lounge, and using his laptop computer, entered data he had gleaned from the convention.*
>
> **John** *allowed the delay "to ruin his day." He tried to read, but he could not concentrate. He frequently glanced at his watch and paced up and down the airport lounge. Furious at the inconvenience, he angrily expressed his frustration to the ticket agent.*

Do you have a constant sense of urgency? Do you notice an underlying feeling of continual anxiety? Are you often hostile toward others? You may be moving toward the more negative Type A personality. Monitor yourself. Are you always feeling rushed, checking your watch and running from project to project, feeling irritated and annoyed with those in your way? Especially be alert to feelings of pent-up rage and dissatisfaction. These emotions impair your resiliency and make you more vulnerable to stress and illness. Take the Personality Type and Job Burnout Checklists presented in Chapter 8 to discover if you are developing negative Type A characteristics. Increasing your awareness of particular responses to stress enables you to make changes. You can restructure a Type A personality: retaining such qualities as enthusiasm for success and high productivity, and reducing such emotions as hostility, anger, and impatience.

Finding Your "Stimulation Comfort" Zone

Even as you work on the variables affecting your ability to cope with stress, it is vital to honor your current level of resilience.

What is the right amount of stimulation for you? Although you can stretch your capacity to manage stress, maintaining wellness also means recognizing your natural comfort zone for stimulation. How big can the storms of life become before you are no longer challenged, but overwhelmed? How calm can the seas be before a peaceful, contented life becomes boring?

You can be over-stimulated or under-stimulated by the demands of life and work. Either too much or too little stimulation leads to stress. The same input—demands, stimulation, change—may be too little or boring for one person, and for another can be too much, causing anxiety and a sense of being overwhelmed. For some, bungee cord jumping is just the ticket. Sailing down through the sky, wind whistling by my ears, clothes flapping, eyes fixed on the rapidly approaching earth, would definitely be over-stimulating for me!

Many people struggle throughout life to find some middle ground between boredom and over-stimulation (Preston, 1993). Try to establish a balance between feeling bored and overwhelmed. The optimal amount of stimulation is based on our personality and the tools we have (and use) to cope with the pressures in our lives. When you find your optimal level of stimulation, you will feel enthusiastic and motivated by life's challenges.

As we have seen, wellness, in addition to learning stress-reducing skills, includes processing past pain and living within the parameters of your current "stimulation comfort" zone.

Creating Your Stress Profile

In the next four chapters you will be given a series of checklists to create your own Stress Profile. Using these self-assessment tools will enable you to then design an effective Wellness Program based on stress reduction activities that fit your personal profile.

Using the checklists, you will assess:

1. Your work stressors. These refer to situations you may or may not be able to change such as a critical supervisor, lack of job security, or a noisy environment.

2. Your stress symptoms. These refer to your physical, emotional, and behavioral responses to job stress.

3. Symptoms for depression and anxiety.

4. Your personality type. You can check to see if you fit a negative Type A personality and/or have reached the point of "burnout" on the job.

5

Measuring Your Work Site Stressors

Peace on earth will come from making peace inside yourself and bringing it with you into the world.

—Stephen C. Paul, *Illuminations*

Now that you understand the basic physiology of stress, and why each person's resilience to stress is different, the next step in bringing wellness to your work is to create your own Stress Profile. Begin by taking an inventory of the stressors in your work life. Stress research has documented a specific correlation between the number and severity of stressors in one's life and the probability of mental or physical illness. Probability of illness can be reduced by learning new mental, emotional, and physical responses to stress, and by training yourself to evoke the relaxation response.

Exactly what is it that stresses you at work? How many and how severe are these stressors? Once you recognize your workplace stressors, you can use the symptoms check-lists to assess the impact of these stressors on your mental and physical health. After identifying your warning signs and symptoms, you can take appropriate preventive action to maintain your wellness at work. Let's first find out how much pressure you are up against.

——— WORK SITE STRESSORS CHECKLIST ———

Rate each of the ten stressors listed below on a scale from one to ten, one for a low impact stressor, ten for a high impact stressor. Under each stressor are some possible variations. Check those that apply to you. You may have some of your own unique variations. You can add these to the list. The purpose is to accurately assess what stresses you the most at work. Rate stressors which have occurred any time during the past year. Total your score.

In scoring the impact of your stressors, use the following scale as a guide.

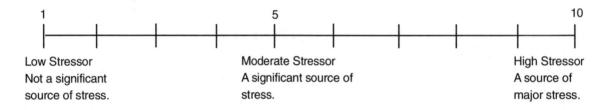

1	5	10
Low Stressor	Moderate Stressor	High Stressor
Not a significant	A significant source of	A source of
source of stress.	stress.	major stress.

Score

_____ 1. I have inharmonious work relationships, such as

☐ uncommunicative coworkers or supervisors

☐ aggressive colleagues or customers

☐ discordant relationship with boss

☐ incompatibility with boss or coworkers

_____ 2. I have little say in the decision-making process, including such examples as

☐ responsibility without much authority

☐ to voice my opinions or feelings would jeopardize my job

☐ not being included in important planning meetings/decisions

☐ my decisions are often challenged or contradicted

_____ 3. My job conflicts with social/family obligations because of

☐ incompatible working hours with spouse/family members' needs

☐ constant shift changes

☐ change in working hours

    ☐ transfer to new office/location

_____ 4. Unpleasant/relatively unsafe work environment or commute such as

    ☐ negative change in working conditions such as decrease in privacy

    ☐ long commute with lots of traffic

    ☐ noisy or hazardous environment

    ☐ uncomfortable environment: poor lighting, recycled air, no windows

    ☐ physical discomfort: long hours sitting or standing

_____ 5. There are uncomfortable aspects about my workload such as

    ☐ deadline pressures

    ☐ information overload

    ☐ decrease in hours and/or income

    ☐ too much or too little work

_____ 6. I am hassled or discriminated against at work due to

    ☐ sex, color, or age

    ☐ religion, politics, or fashion

    ☐ appearance, life style, or values

_____ 7. I don't feel adequately appreciated for the work I do because

    ☐ inadequate pay for amount of work

    ☐ others take credit for my ideas

    ☐ boss is highly critical and rarely says thanks

    ☐ there is little or no opportunity for advancement

_____ 8. I do not have job security because of

    ☐ recession-related business reorganization—lay-offs, mergers, bankruptcy

    ☐ ambiguity of job description

    ☐ my over-qualification or under-qualification for the job

    ☐ highly competitive and shrinking job market

_____ 9. My job, or my job description, has changed or is changing due to

    ☐ promotion

☐   demotion

☐   retirement

☐   change to a different line of work

_____ 10. I do not feel proud or rewarded by my work because

☐   it is tedious and treated as trivial at work

☐   it isn't the type of work I most want to do or isn't in my field of interest

☐   there are conflicts with my values and beliefs

☐   my friends/family don't respect what I do

_____ **Total Score**

Job Stress Score Rating:

10–29	Low
30–59	Moderate
60–80	High
81–100	Intense

—— INTERPRETING YOUR RESULTS, CHOOSING YOUR BATTLES ——

Now that you have rated your level of workplace stressors, including those that apply to your unique situation, take time to evaluate the information.

Choosing Your Battles

Review the list and categorize the stressors according to those you can change and those that you can't change.

Focus your time and creativity on those stressors you can change. For example, what is your contribution to a discordant relationship with the boss or incompatibility with a coworker? Or, as another example, do you need to learn to be more assertive regarding deadline pressures or unpaid overtime work?

Are some of your stressors ones that you cannot realistically change? For example, a long commute with lots of traffic, incompatible working hours with your spouse, or a hazardous work environment?

Acknowledge those stressors you can't do anything about and "let go" or reconcile yourself with this lack of control. This is a challenging task, and perhaps a life-long project, but there are skills you can learn in order to let go more easily.

Review your list of stressors and circle those that are a significant or major source of stress (5–10 rating). Under the following columns categorize these stressors into those you feel you can change and those you feel you can't change.

Stressors I Can Change   *Stressors I Cannot Change*

_____   _____

_____   _____

_____   _____

_____   _____

Choosing Your Response

Part II presents ways to address your work stressors. You can choose relaxation skills, cognitive skills, nutrition and exercise, and communication skills to cope with your stressors. You will be referred back to your stressors to see if a solution that is suggested applies to your situation. For example, if you rated #1 high, in harmonious work relationships, you will need to look closely at the chapter on feelings and communications. If you get highly stressed by deadline pressures which cannot be changed (#5), you may need to focus on relaxation skills or changing your thinking patterns.

Now that you recognize what your worksite stressors are, use the next chapter to measure your physical, emotional, and behavioral responses to your stressors.

6

Measuring Your Stress Responses

*Fortunately, we can change how we perceive ourselves and how
we relate to the stressors in our lives. We can acquire the skills
and the resources to deal with stress as a challenge and as a
learning opportunity.*

—Patricia Norris quoted in
Healers on Healing

Some people express stress primarily in their bodies, as disease. Others manifest stress psychologically, as depression, anxiety, or a multitude of other emotional forms. Still others act out stress behaviorally. Some people manifest a combination of these responses.

Stress management works best by treating both the symptoms and the cause. For example, if you have ulcers, make the medical and diet changes indicated, and also alleviate the ulcer-contributing anxiety. Treatment of physical symptoms alone may bring temporary results, but the underlying anxiety will surely express itself again—either as the same problem or something else.

The next step in creating your Stress Profile is to evaluate the relative intensity of your stress and to know how you respond to stress physically, psychologically, and behaviorally. After each checklist is information to help you evaluate your symptoms.

——— *PHYSICAL RESPONSES CHECKLIST* ———

Using the following scale of frequency, circle the number that best describes the frequency of the symptoms that you experience due to stress. Then total your score.

	Never	Seldom (less than once a month)	Infrequent (once a month)	Occasional (more than once a month)	Very often (more than once a week)	Constant
Cardiovascular						
Rapid, shallow breathing	0	1	2	3	4	5
Tightness in chest	0	1	2	3	4	5
Heart pounding	0	1	2	3	4	5
High blood pressure	0	1	2	3	4	5
Vascular						
Migraine headache	0	1	2	3	4	5
Tension headache	0	1	2	3	4	5
Clammy hands/feet	0	1	2	3	4	5
Gastrointestinal						
Diarrhea	0	1	2	3	4	5
Constipation	0	1	2	3	4	5
Burping	0	1	2	3	4	5
Flatulence (gas)	0	1	2	3	4	5
Colitis	0	1	2	3	4	5
Indigestion	0	1	2	3	4	5
Ulcers	0	1	2	3	4	5
Muscular						
Backache	0	1	2	3	4	5
Neck pain	0	1	2	3	4	5
Muscle tension	0	1	2	3	4	5
Jaw pain/tension	0	1	2	3	4	5
Neurological						
Tics/tremors	0	1	2	3	4	5
Dizziness	0	1	2	3	4	5
Dry mouth	0	1	2	3	4	5

Skin

Skin rash	0	1	2	3	4	5
Acne	0	1	2	3	4	5

Immune System

Frequent colds	0	1	2	3	4	5
Increase in allergies	0	1	2	3	4	5

Other

Increase in the urge to urinate	0	1	2	3	4	5
Menstrual distress/PMS	0	1	2	3	4	5
Asthma	0	1	2	3	4	5
Fatigue	0	1	2	3	4	5
Sleeping difficulties	0	1	2	3	4	5

_____ **Total Score**

Score Interpretation:
0-9 You're doing great!
10-20 Comfortable handling of stress.
21-34 Could sharpen coping skills.
35-70 Time for changes.

Over 70 Get help now. You are highly stressed.

Your score may be skewed because your pain is not due to stress, but has a physical cause, such as an accident, surgery, or other cause. Adjust your score downward if this is the case. For example, if your skin rash is due to poison oak, do not assign a number to skin rash.

Evaluating Your Physical Responses to Stress

Review the checklist and look for symptoms that you rated 4 or 5. If your score for each item in a particular biological system is three or more, see your doctor. Take special care if stress seems to be affecting your cardiovascular system or immune system.

Use Part II to address your symptoms. For example, if you are experiencing frequent stress in your gastrointestinal system as stomach pain or digestive disorders, focus on the nutrition suggestions in Part II.

If you indicated muscle tension, focus on the chapters on deep relaxation and exercise.

Your stress-related physical symptoms can be reduced by improved self-care. A healthy diet, cardiovascular exercise, gentle stretching, and practice of relaxation skills will reduce your symptoms. All of these are taught in Part II.

——— PSYCHOLOGICAL RESPONSES CHECKLIST ———

Psychological responses to stress can be loosely divided into low energy or high energy emotional responses. With a high energy response such as rage, there is the emotional imbalance of too much charge or intensity. With a low energy response such as depression, there is a lack of normal vitality or energy.

Using the following scale, circle the number which best describes the frequency of your experience of the following stress indicators, and total your score.

	Never	Seldom (less than once a month)	Infrequent (once a month)	Occasional (more than once a month)	Very often (more than once a week)	Constant
Low Energy Responses						
I feel depressed at work, or when thinking about work.	0	1	2	3	4	5
I feel a sense of hopelessness regarding my job.	0	1	2	3	4	5
I feel powerless regarding my work situation.	0	1	2	3	4	5
I feel of little personal value at work.	0	1	2	3	4	5
I am bored at work.	0	1	2	3	4	5
I am fearful of someone or something at work.	0	1	2	3	4	5
High Energy Responses						
I am angry at someone at work or over a work situation.	0	1	2	3	4	5
I feel irritable at work.	0	1	2	3	4	5
I feel resentful toward a person at work or a work situation.	0	1	2	3	4	5
I feel a sense of hostility regarding work.	0	1	2	3	4	5
I am anxious regarding deadlines or work load.	0	1	2	3	4	5
I am anxious regarding a relationship at work.	0	1	2	3	4	5
I am frustrated regarding a work situation or relationship.	0	1	2	3	4	5

I am restless at work.   0   1   2   3   4   5

_____ **Total Score**

Score Interpretation:
0-15   Comfortable handling stress.
16-25   Could sharpen coping skills.
26-45   Time for changes.
Over 46   Take action and get help now.

Evaluating Your Psychological Responses to Stress

If you indicated more frequent low energy psychological response solutions to stress, you will want to focus on solutions that take very little effort and at the same time they increase one's energy. For example, good posture and breathing techniques increase the body's supply of oxygen (energy) but take very little exertion.

In Part II, practice breathing exercises, gentle physical exercises, and reevaluate your perceptions of yourself and your work situation using the cognitive skills and communications chapters. Use the next chapter to assess yourself for depression.

If you indicated more frequent high energy psychological response solutions, you may have too much energy to focus on the more subtle tools of stress management. In Part II, focus on the benefits of physical exercise. You may also need to make diet changes such as reducing caffeine. Use the next chapter to assess yourself for anxiety. If you think you might be a Type A personality go through the Type A Personality Checklist in Chapter 8.

—— *BEHAVIORAL RESPONSES CHECKLIST* ——

Circle the number that best describes the frequency of the following symptoms. Then total your score.

	Never	Seldom (less than once a month)	Infrequent (once a month)	Occasional (more than once a month)	Very often (more than once a week)	Constant
Gum chewing	0	1	2	3	4	5
Teeth grinding	0	1	2	3	4	5
Procrastinating	0	1	2	3	4	5
Irregular eating habits	0	1	2	3	4	5
Clenching fists	0	1	2	3	4	5
Nail biting	0	1	2	3	4	5

	Never	Seldom (less than once a month)	Infrequent (once a month)	Occasional (more than once a month)	Very often (more than once a week)	Constant
Rapid/loud talking	0	1	2	3	4	5
Emotionally overreacting	0	1	2	3	4	5
Failing to complete projects	0	1	2	3	4	5
Doing several things simultaneously	0	1	2	3	4	5

_____ **Total Score**

Score Interpretation:

0-7	Comfortable handling stress
8-15	Could sharpen stress reducing skills
16-25	Time for changes
26-50	Take stress management action now

Evaluating Your Behavioral Responses to Stress

Even if you sailed through the checklists for Physical and Psychological Responses to Stress, you may have "flunked" the Behavioral Responses Checklist. Often people with few psychological or physical indicators of stress score high on the behavioral checklist. Behavioral responses stem from numerous causes. Let's look at a few possibilities.

Your upbringing could have caused you to suppress emotions, resulting in pent-up feelings being expressed behaviorally rather than emotionally. Often parents demand behaviors from their children that are not congruent with the child's experience. Many parents demand that Johnny or Suzy curb expression of their legitimate feelings.

> *"Johnny, stop crying. Big boys don't cry."*
> *"Suzy, be nice. Give Mrs. Van Humphrys a hug."*
> *"Benny, don't be ridiculous. Do you want people to think you're a scaredy-cat? Jump in the water now, or I'll throw you in."*
> *"Janie, that's stupid for you to feel hurt. There are a million other guys out there for you."*

These statements and hundreds like them often cause children to hide their feelings or question the legitimacy of their emotions. The child that is now an adult continues to suppress emotions. One of my clients provides a perfect example. Mary, a principal at a junior high school, could not express or trust her feelings. She had burn scars on the inside of her wrists from doing dishes in water that her mother insisted was not too hot. This experience resulted in nightly teeth grinding and a subtle distancing in relationships.

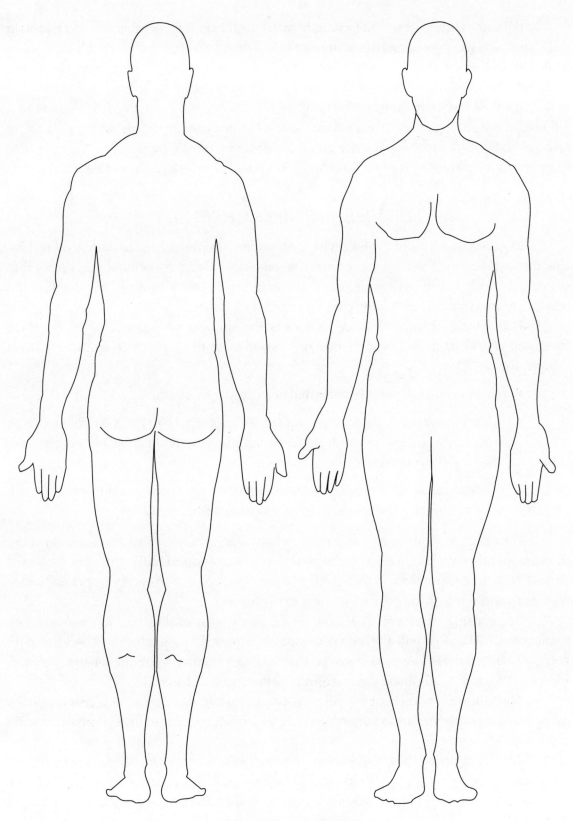

Visual Stress Checklist

For some families there is a tacit understanding that family members should maintain the "family image" by acting happy in front of outsiders. Other families find it best not to deal with feelings at all. Parents in these families do not show affection to each other, and topics of conversation are always about *doing* rather than *feeling*.

If any of these situations sound familiar, you may not be in touch with your feelings, although your feelings may be expressed through your behavior. Focus on the chapter on feelings and communications at work and the chapter on reframing your thinking patterns to become more aware of your feelings and learn healthy ways to express them.

——— THE VISUAL STRESS CHECKLIST ———

My clients have used the following deceptively simple technique with good results. Creative expression of your stress symptoms increases awareness of how you respond to stress and subtly encourages your participation in the recovery process. It's also fun and relaxing to do. You will need some colored pencils or markers.

Using the preceding drawing, fill in the symptoms you identified in the three foregoing checklists as follows. Include only your most troublesome (significant) stress symptoms:

- *Circle* each of your body parts that are affected by stress.

- *Color* in your psychological responses with colors that best describe your feelings. You may also color over a label. For example, you might color red (anger) over the label, "clenched jaw."

- *Write* in the word or words that best describes your behavioral responses, such as gum chewing, clenching fists, or procrastinating.

For example, Bonnie, an elementary school teacher, found that she reacts to stress most frequently with a tight neck, feelings of powerlessness, and nail biting. On the Visual Stress Checklist she put a red X on the back of the neck, colored the body from head to toe with gray, and wrote "biting my nails" next to the fingers.

Recognizing ways you typically exhibit stress will enable you to choose stress-reduction activities that will alleviate your stress symptoms. The symptoms checklists help you pinpoint your responses to stress so that you can fashion a comprehensive personal Wellness Program to eliminate the undesirable effects of job stress.

The following two chapters will help you to further develop your Stress Profile by pinpointing whether you are experiencing to a greater degree some of the symptoms already discussed.

After completing these checklists on depression, anxiety, personality, and job burnout return to this chapter and add the most significant symptoms to your Visual Stress Checklist. For example, you might write insomnia next to your head or color your heart blue for depression.

7

Assessing Depression and Anxiety

Focusing attention and energy to positive aspects in one's life is a "healing technique" in and of itself.

—Jo Ann Cannon,
What's Right with Your Life?

Do you feel guilty because you can't get out of bed in the morning? Do you find you can't muster enthusiasm? Do you find it difficult to concentrate? Perhaps you are constantly "on edge." Rest assured, these are symptoms of disease rather than a sign of your being lazy or dull, and you may be one of the approximately 35 million Americans who are afflicted with moderate depression or anxiety—the two most common psychological responses to stress (Regier et al., 1984).

Depression and anxiety are illnesses, and they have specific, treatable symptoms. Many people suffering from anxiety or depression do not recognize they are ill, and their belief that something is "wrong" with them compounds their illness.

Not everyone who has stress symptoms has a depressive or anxiety disorder. If you have suffered from a number of stress-related symptoms on a frequent basis for a prolonged period without treatment, you may have developed depression or an anxiety disorder. If this is true, you may need to get professional help in addition to using the stress reduction techniques in this book. See Part III for information for finding an appropriate counselor.

It is reassuring to learn what the symptoms are, and helpful to understand what the impact on society is. The National Institute for Occupational Safety and Health, the principal federal agency concerned with work-related hazards, has called work-related psychological disorders "a leading occupational health problem" (Sauter et al., 1990). Over 75 percent of all general medical care practice is for people plagued with stress-related symptoms, and the majority of these are job-related (Wallace, 1992).

In 1978 the President's Commission on Mental Health recommended devising improved methods for measuring the prevalence of mental disorders among Americans and their use of mental health services. The National Institute for Mental Health responded with a landmark, comprehensive and unprecedented study based on approximately 20,000 people in five communities across the United States (Regier et al., 1993). NIMH figures for the adult civilian population of the United States in 1990 show the following:

- Anxiety or depression comprise over 80 percent of all mental or addictive disorders.

- One in every four civilian adults suffers from anxiety or depression.

- Less than 30 percent of those with anxiety disorders receive professional help.

- Only 50 percent of those experiencing major depression receive professional help.

- Only 40 percent of those with dysthymia (more than two years of chronic mild depressive symptoms) receive professional help (Regier, 1993).

The following checklists will help clarify whether you are experiencing depression or anxiety.

If you are anxious or depressed, you need to take your stress seriously and take action immediately. After each of the following assessments, there is a list of suggestions to put into practice now. However, to learn and develop new responses to stress, you will need to go through the techniques in the book and practice them until you feel comfortable with them and then put them into a program you are committed to using on a regular basis. Awareness is the first step. Change takes time and consistent practice. It may take at least a month of regular practice before you experience significant relief from your anxiety or depression.

——— DEPRESSION CHECKLIST ———

Depression is the most common response to repeated and untreated stress. You may or may not be aware of the specific stressor(s) causing your depression. Often there is no precipitating event that you can pinpoint. Check those symptoms that apply to you (*DSM IV*, 1994):

_____ 1. More often than not, I am depressed for most of the day.

_____ 2. I have lost my enthusiasm for most activities.

_____ 3. I am having problems sleeping (insomnia or hypersomnia).

_____ 4. I feel tired or fatigued most of the time.

_____ 5. I have a low opinion of myself. I usually feel worthless or guilty.

_____ 6. I am unable to concentrate. I am indecisive.

_____ 7. I feel overwhelmed; I feel a sense of hopelessness.

_____ 8. I feel either edgy or slowed down.

_____ 9. I have suicidal thoughts. I don't want to be here any more.

_____ 10. I have had a significant weight gain or loss not due to dieting.

If you are experiencing any one of these symptoms, it is time for action. If you are having suicidal thoughts, immediately call your doctor.

First Aid for Depression

1. Turn to friends or family for support. Don't isolate yourself. See the chapter on social support and Part III on professional services.

2. Initiate an exercise program or sport. Take a walk during your lunch break with a friend.

3. Reduce alcohol consumption. Alcohol is a depressant.

4. Pamper yourself with a massage, a movie, or a day to yourself to do whatever you want. Even pampering yourself once a month can make a world of difference. Your well-being is worth the extra cost of a babysitter.

5. Avoid overeating. Especially reduce your sugar and fat intake.

6. Avoid financial overload. Prioritize your expenditures or seek professional help from a financial consultant.

7. See Part II for additional skills to combat depression. If you have low self-esteem, focus on the chapters on reframing your thinking patterns and communication. Continue your education on stress reduction through classes in your local community or Wellness Programs at work.

If your symptoms continue unchanged for over a week, or if all of the above suggestions sound too difficult or unappealing, see your doctor.

———— ANXIETY CHECKLIST ————

The following are symptoms of anxiety. You may experience some mild depressive symptoms from the Depression Checklist along with the anxiety symptoms described below. This is common, especially since there is an overlap of symptoms. This checklist helps you identify signals that indicate you are on overload. Check the symptoms that apply to you (*DSM IV*, 1994):

_____ 1. I often feel shaky or tremble.

_____ 2. I experience muscular tension or aches.

_____ 3. I feel edgy and keyed up.

_____ 4. I am easily tired.

_____ 5. I feel restless most of the time.

_____ 6. I am startled easily.

_____ 7. I feel irritable.

_____ 8. I have problems falling or staying asleep.

_____ 9. I have difficulty concentrating. I keep forgetting things.

_____ 10. I keep worrying all the time. I dwell on problems.

Nine Anxiety Busters

1. Learn how to set limits—say "no" to certain activities and people. See the chapter on communication skills. Pare down your agenda so that you have more time for activities meaningful to you.

2. Delegate or share responsibilities or workload when appropriate. Recognize that you cannot do everything.

3. Learn how to prioritize.

4. Take enough "space" or time alone—in nature, if possible.

5. Allow time for personal creative expression—especially through writing, art, music, or dance.

6. Give yourself permission to relax, by reading, daydreaming, playing board games or cards, stretching out in the sun, or curling up in a hammock.

7. Revise your expectations of yourself and of others. Be realistic, so that you don't feel guilty or agitated when a project isn't completed by an arbitrary or unrealistic deadline.

8. Cut down on caffeine. Consumption of only two cups of coffee *contributes* to feelings of anxiety; more than two cups of coffee *creates* feelings/symptoms of anxiety. See Appendix A for a chart on the caffeine content of certain foods and beverages.

9. See Part II for other means of combating anxiety, especially the chapters on physical activities and relaxation skills.

8

Assessing Personality Type and Job Burnout

One of the keys to reducing stress isn't just removing negative experiences from your life, but adding positive ones.

—Berkeley Health Letter Associates

Is your harried life style causing you distress because you've become addicted to work, unable to slow down? Do you find you are driving away family, friends, and coworkers due to your excessively competitive style? Are you hostile, edgy, and unhappy? Now is the time for honest self-appraisal. The following checklists are designed to help you become more aware of your stress-induced behavior and emotions.

An important factor in stress management is to recognize your personality type, which is defined by specific behaviors and emotions. Type B personalities—people who do not have a sense of time urgency—are easy-going, congenial, unhurried, and content—are less prone to stress than Type A personalities.

Type A personalities—people who are ambitious, driven to be the best in everything they do, enthusiastic, and hard-working—are often high achievers. But they need to recognize that these traits make them vulnerable to stress and can erode into unhealthy, negative behaviors and emotions that contribute to job burnout.

To start mark where you see yourself on the Type A to Type B continuum below (Tubesing, 1990). This is an informal method of quickly evaluating your personality type. Then compare with your actual personality type scores.

100% Type A   50/50 Type A/B   100% Type B

I_____I_____I_____I_____I_____I_____I_____I_____I_____I

———— NEGATIVE TYPE A PERSONALITY CHECKLIST ————

The following checklist will help you assess whether you are developing negative Type A tendencies. Using the following scale of frequency, circle the number that best describes the frequency of the symptoms that you experience. Then total your score.

	Never	Seldom (less than once a month)	Occasional (one to four times a month)	Often (more than once a week)	Usual, constant
Sense of Time					
I walk, eat, move rapidly.	0	1	2	3	4
I interrupt or finish the speech of others.	0	1	2	3	4
Waiting in line irritates me.	0	1	2	3	4
I say "Yes . . . yes, yes" or "Uh-huh . . . uh-huh" when others are speaking.	0	1	2	3	4
I am infuriated by slow drivers in front of me.	0	1	2	3	4
I do several things simultaneously.	0	1	2	3	4
I feel guilty or edgy when relaxing; or, I am unable to relax.	0	1	2	3	4
I am impatient with delays and take over if others are too slow.	0	1	2	3	4
I work feverishly; I am obsessed with deadlines.	0	1	2	3	4
I feel rushed and pressured.	0	1	2	3	4
I drive myself, ignoring physical limitations.	0	1	2	3	4
Feelings of Self-Worth					
My success in life is based on my success at work.	0	1	2	3	4

I evaluate my success at work only in terms of dollars earned, projects completed, products sold, or similar objective standards.	0	1	2	3	4
I am very competitive; I play to win, not for enjoyment.	0	1	2	3	4

Generalized Feelings

I experience an unrelenting sense of tension/anxiety.	0	1	2	3	4
I feel hostile toward people.	0	1	2	3	4
I lack a sense of inner peace or contentment.	0	1	2	3	4

_____   **Total Score:**

Score Interpretation:

0-17	Few, if any, negative Type A tendencies
18-25	Moderate negative Type A personality
26-50	Full-Blown negative Type A personality

——— *Type B Personality Checklist* ———

Fill in the number that best describes the frequency of your behaviors and attitudes. Then total your score.

	Never	Seldom (less than once a month)	Occasional (one to four times a month)	Often (more than once a week)	Usual, constant
Sense of Time					
I can work without agitation, even under pressure.	0	1	2	3	4
I enjoy relaxing, and the poetic side of life.	0	1	2	3	4
I do not get anxious from unexpected interruptions.	0	1	2	3	4
I feel comfortable leaving tasks undone while I relax.	0	1	2	3	4
Feelings of Self-Worth					
My value is not exclusively based on work achievements.	0	1	2	3	4
I enjoy sports and games for fun, not to win or prove my superiority.	0	1	2	3	4

	Never	Seldom (less than once a month)	Occasional (one to four times a month)	Often (more than once a week)	Usual, constant
Generalized Feelings					
I am relaxed and easy going.	0	1	2	3	4
I am not driven or highly ambitious.	0	1	2	3	4

_____   **Total Score:**

Score Interpretation:

0-10	I have few, if any, Type B tendencies
11-25	Moderate Type B personality
26-50	Full-Blown Type B personality

Evaluating Your Responses

Obviously, if you have developed more of the negative Type A personality you are more prone to stress than someone who is a Type B or a mixed type A/B. Type A personalities can learn to improve coping skills. One of the most effective means of becoming a more healthy Type A personality is to practice some form of relaxation. Meditation, yoga, biofeedback, or deep relaxation along with improved communication skills and modified cognitive and emotional responses to stress can modify the negative Type A personality from a driven, hostile, and impatient person into a healthy, pleasant, and happy Type A personality (Zeff, 1981).

———— JOB BURNOUT CHECKLIST ————

You are a candidate for job burnout if stress at work combined with your personality type creates negative behaviors and feelings. Usually job burnout develops out of intensification of the stress load. The original positive qualities of hard work, enthusiasm, and ambition have dissolved into the frustration of unmet expectations, cynicism, and pessimism (Klarreich, 1990). Check those symptoms that apply to you:

_____ I feel exhausted physically and/or emotionally when I am at work.

_____ I have lost interest regarding work or coworkers.

_____ I am pessimistic about my work situation.

_____ I have a negative view regarding the future of my career.

_____ I distrust coworkers and company management. I am cynical regarding relationships at work.

_____ I am abdicating my responsibilities at work.

_____ There is a change in my eating and/or sleeping pattern.

_____ I am irritable and on edge, especially at work.

_____ I feel depleted and depressed, especially at work.

SCORE: If you have checked four or more of the above symptoms, your depression can be the result of job burnout.

Evaluating Your Responses

If you are experiencing job burnout, tailor the techniques presented in Part II to match your profile. Choose appropriate relaxation skills to balance your driving work ethic. Take up aerobic exercise to release stored tension. Practice the cognitive reframing exercises to modify your time urgency perceptions. It is especially important to learn to value yourself as a human *being*, not just a human *doing*!

In the next chapter, which concludes Part I, you will compile the information from the checklists above with the results of the checklists you completed on your worksite stressors and responses to stress to create your Stress Profile.

9

Compiling Your Stress Profile

Setting goals and working toward them fuel creativity and invention. The desire to change things activates progress.

—Joan Borysenko, *Minding the Body, Mending the Mind*

You are now armed with vital information! Having completed the preceding checklists, you know:

- How stress negatively impacts health

- What conditions at work stress you

- Your particular physical, emotional, and behavioral responses to stress

- Your personality type

- Whether you are experiencing job burnout

- Whether you are suffering from anxiety or depression

To compile your Stress Profile go back over your checklists in Chapters 5 through 8 and use that information to fill in the following chart.

——— *MY STRESS PROFILE* ———

My most significant work site stressors:

Use your checklist from Chapter 5 and elaborate as desired.

1. _____

2. _____

3. _____

4. _____

5. _____

6. _____

My most frequent, troublesome stress symptoms:

List those you experience most often or most desire to reduce. Refer to checklists in Chapter 6 if needed.

Physical:

1. _____

2. _____

3. _____

Emotional/Psychological:

1. _____

2. _____

3. _____

Behavioral:

1. _____

2. _____

3. _____

Anxiety and depression symptoms:

List your most frequent prolonged, intense symptoms from Chapter 7:

Depression: Anxiety:

1. _____   1. _____

2. _____   2. _____

3. _____   3. _____

4. _____   4. _____

My personality type:

Indicate personality type and specific behaviors/attitudes you desire to modify. Refer to Chapter 8 if needed.

Type: _____

Behaviors:_____

1. _____

2. _____

3. _____

My level of burnout:

Indicate number of burnout signs and which ones you want to address.

Number: _____

Signs: _____

1. _____

2. _____

3. _____

With your personal Stress Profile in hand, you are ready to begin Part II and learn which techniques you want to adopt to design your Wellness Program. Each stress management technique in Part II counteracts a variety of stress symptoms. Learn and practice all of the techniques in Part II before deciding which ones seem to be the most effective for your specific stressors and symptoms.

Each chapter describes the techniques and how to use them, offering case examples of their application to typical stressful work situations. At the end of each chapter you are invited to complete an exercise demonstrating how you could use the techniques in your own work life.

At the end of Part II are guidelines to formulate your overall Wellness Program. It will consist of the stress management techniques you have chosen to combine and use on a regular basis.

Part II

ELEMENTS OF A WELLNESS PROGRAM

10

Relaxation Therapy and Your Wellness Program—An Overview

An early morning walk is a blessing for the whole day.

—Henry David Thoreau

The heart of any wellness program is conscious relaxation skills. You need no special equipment or lengthy courses of study. These skills are helping many people to overcome the pain and expense of high-stress existence and to regain the joy of living. Surely relaxation skills will be one of the great legacies of our time! The relaxation skills presented in this section are the premier tools of stress management. They will enable you to gain control over physiological responses to psychosocial stressors.

Through relaxation skills you train your body to respond differently to stress. When you first perceive an experience as threatening, *and for as long as the anxiety continues,* your body will experience increased heart rate, blood pressure, and respiration, along with shallow or irregular breath, tense muscles, and a slowing of the digestive process. This is the stress response. The purpose of eliciting the relaxation response is to reduce these negative effects from an overstimulated sympathetic system (Benson, 1976). A learned relaxation response allows the body to switch from the flight-or-fight mode into a rest-and-repair mode. Dr. Herbert Benson, Harvard cardiologist, author, and researcher, coined the term "relaxation response" to refer to the condition in which the heart slows down, the blood pressure drops, the muscles relax, the breath slows and deepens, the digestive process improves and the brain waves go into a mode related to peace and calmness. It is natural for the body to change from one mode to the other in response to the exigencies of the moment, but many people get stuck in a high-gear stress response and become increasingly unable to relax. By increasing control of your physiological reactions to stress, you will improve your ability to handle life's pressures and disappointments.

Relaxation skills are particularly helpful for those experiencing symptoms of anxiety. No matter what your stress symptoms, learning how to shift from your high-gear stress response and relax correctly by eliciting the relaxation response can reduce your stress symptoms.

You may feel relief immediately, or it may take as much as a month before noticing relief. Although success is not guaranteed, most people have been greatly helped by mastering these techniques.

When done correctly, each of the relaxation skills elicits the relaxation response. Practice all of them. *Practice each technique until you have mastered it.* Once you can elicit the relaxation response, you may prefer to continue with just one form of practice. Choose one or more which best fits your schedule, life style, or preference, but *be sure to choose one in which you actually elicit the relaxation response.* The literature on stress management provides no clear-cut evidence as to the superiority of one method of relaxation over another in eliciting the relaxation response or reducing stress symptoms. Choose those most effective for you.

Initially, daily practice in a quiet setting is best. But once you have experienced the reduction of stress symptoms, integrate the techniques into your daily work routine in short-form and use them whenever you are in a stressful work situation. You can learn to relax physiologically in the midst of stress. Relaxation training allows you to relax or to gear up appropriately.

Limits and Contraindications

Occasionally, some people may experience "relaxation-induced" anxiety. During the relaxation response, there may be a surfacing of previously suppressed or unconscious feelings. Because usual defense mechanisms are lower, previously hidden (subconscious) thoughts and emotions which cause anxiety may be revealed. This is a rare response, but can be welcomed as an opportunity for deeper self-understanding of the subconscious issues causing surface anxiety. If you do respond to the relaxation techniques with increased anxiety, have a therapist assist you in integrating your newly gained, personal insights, and guide you in practicing the relaxation training. After learning the techniques, Part III provides information on finding appropriate professional help.

There are no known contraindications to relaxation, meditation, or biofeedback, but if you are on medication with major systemic effects, such as antihypertensive drugs, thyroid medication, or insulin, consult your physician to monitor any physiological changes. Similarly, if you have high blood pressure, Harvard cardiologist Dr. Benson and others state that, no matter how encouraging the results, no one should treat himself for high blood pressure or other diseases by regularly eliciting the relaxation response unless under the guidance of a physician *who will routinely monitor your blood pressure (or other system under medication) to make sure it is adequately controlled* (Benson, 1976).

The following four chapters on Conscious Breathing, Deep Relaxation, Meditation, and Biofeedback present techniques specifically designed to elicit the relaxation response.

After learning how to elicit the relaxation response the remaining chapters in Part IV provide techniques and exercises to further ruduce job stress through physical activity, good nutrition, social support, self-care, clear thinking, and sound communication—the main ingredients to a strong, effective Wellness Program. Use the exercises provided in each chapter and practice the techniques until you have mastered them. At the conclusion of Part II, you will combine the techniques most effective for you into your own Wellness Program.

11

Conscious Breathing

Healthy breathing techniques are easy to learn and can have profound effects on one's life.

—The Center for Applied Psychophysiology,
The Menninger Clinic

Proper breathing is the cornerstone of stress management. Although we all breathe, few of us retain the habit of full, natural breathing we had when we were young. Conscious breathing means relearning how to breathe more deeply and completely. In addition, your breath directly reflects your emotional state. When you are calm, your breathing is deep and slow. When you are feeling stressed, your breathing changes. For example, when you are nervous about an upcoming interview your breath is shallow and erratic. Conscious breathing allows you to take charge of your breathing patterns, change the rhythm, and thereby affect your emotions. Proper breathing converts fatigue into vitality, and restlessness into calmness.

The Menninger Clinic, the renowned medical clinic and psychophysiology research and educational center in Topeka, Kansas, has documented the extremely powerful effects of breathing on body functions. Their research shows that learning to be aware of your breathing and practicing healthier breathing techniques is an important step toward gaining optimal health and self-regulation over the physical and mental effects of the stress response (Menninger Clinic, n.d.).

Conscious breathing exercises, done correctly, will:

1. Bring you into the present moment.

2. Affect your mood.

3. Increase the flow of oxygen.

4. Quiet your mind.

5. Reduce physical tension.

6. Improve your general physical health.

Using Breath to Focus on the Present

With conscious breathing, as opposed to normal or unconscious breathing, you mentally take charge of a function that usually occurs subconsciously, and do it with present awareness. Stress is essentially anxiety over a *past or future* stressor. Think about what is stressful in your life: does it have to do with an event which happened yesterday, or is it about an upcoming situation? Even if the stress is chronic, as in a job lay-off, the worry is still really focused on past or projected future events—in anger over why you *were* laid off, or whether you *will lose* your car or house to creditors, or in concern regarding *upcoming* interviews. Placing your attention on your present breath immediately reduces your stress.

——— EXPERIENCE THE BREATH-FEELING LINK ———

Have you ever noticed how different your breath is when you are depressed as compared to when you are happy? You can readily demonstrate to yourself the profound difference. Use the following exercise to explore your breathing patterns and also to discover where in your body you hold your emotions.

1. Sit comfortably with your eyes closed and take several slow, deep breaths. Consciously relax your body, starting at your feet and progressing to your head. Take several minutes to relax. Make any adjustments to be comfortable. Then take three to four minutes for each of the following visualizations.

2. Think about an aspect of your life which gives you pleasure or satisfaction, for example, walking with a friend. Imagine who is there or what you would be doing or saying. Allow yourself to experience this part of your life vividly. Take a moment to step back and observe your breath and how your muscles feel. Are you breathing more deeply? Are your shoulders relaxed? Let yourself enjoy these feelings for a few minutes.

3. Now focus on a segment of your life in which you feel tension, stress, or anger: a circumstance which leaves you frustrated, either with yourself or someone else.

For example, your car pool arrives 20 minutes late. Take a moment to experience this part of your life, and then observe your breath and any body part you may be tensing. Has your breath changed? How? Is your jaw clenched? Are your shoulders tense? Your stomach tight? Inhale, and then as you exhale, let go of your focus on this situation in your life, and relax your body.

4. Now focus on a segment of your life which gives you peace, for example, watching the sunset or listening to calming music. Note the change in your breath, the response of your muscles and posture. The slowing of your breath and the softening of your muscles reflect the tranquility you are experiencing.

Just as your breath reflects your mood, you can powerfully influence your mood by consciously changing the rhythm of your breath. Your sympathetic nervous system's flight-or-fight response is stimulated by the erratic and shallow breathing typical of the corresponding anxious emotional condition. When stressed, people tend to constrict the chest or hold the breath, exacerbating the stress response. By changing your breathing pattern, you can increase the flow of oxygen, balance the autonomic nervous system, cleanse the lymphatic system, maximize exchange of carbon dioxide and oxygen, and decrease anxiety and tension!

Conscious Breathing Techniques

Take time to practice the first exercise, The Abdominal Breath, and the second, The Complete Breath, in depth. These first two exercises are the basics. The last two are variations for extra calming and extra energy. Often people tell me they know how to do these exercises, but in observing them it is clear they don't do them correctly, nor are they obtaining their full benefits. I explain two ways to practice—lying on your back and on your hands and knees. If you experiment and practice *both* ways at home, then it will be easy to breathe abdominally at work, while commuting to and from work, or in conjunction with the other stress reduction exercises. After these exercises, you will be given some specific suggestions of how and when you can use the techniques to reduce stress on the job and an opportunity to come up with your own applications.

—— THE ABDOMINAL BREATH ——

Practice this exercise (also called diaphragmatic breathing) if you are experiencing any stress symptoms. If you hold your tension in the abdominal area, this exercise will be especially beneficial for you.

The abdominal breath is the way you naturally breathe when completely relaxed. The upper portion of the chest and the ribs remains passive while the abdominal area is active. Poor posture, chronic tension in our abdominal muscles, and poor breathing habits override this natural rhythm. The flow of oxygen to the lower part of the lungs is reduced when the abdominal muscles are tense, and assimilation and digestion are inhibited.

By breathing abdominally you not only quiet the mind, but also give a healthy internal massage by the up and down movement of the diaphragm to the organs and tissues of the abdominal area. By breathing abdominally you are activating the parasympathetic side (relaxation side) of your autonomic nervous system.

Dr. Patricia Norris, clinical director of the Biofeedback and Psychophysiology Center at the Menninger Clinic, declares, "I have come to believe that I would choose correct diaphragmatic breathing if we had to share only one tool or technique for maximally improving physical health" (Norris, 1989a).

1. To develop your ability to breathe abdominally, begin by getting a small book and stretching out on your back on the floor. Place the book on your navel.

2. Push the book up toward the ceiling with your abdominal muscles as much as feels comfortable, and then pull the abdominal muscles in, lowering the book closer to the floor. Repeat several times to clarify which muscles you are using.

3. Inhale slowly and deeply through your nose and *relax* the muscles out rather than pushing them out.

4. Exhale through your nose, lowering the book.

5. Keep breathing and watch the book rise and fall in rhythm to the muscle movement. Inhale, letting your muscles relax and moving the book toward the ceiling; exhale, letting your muscles contract and moving the book toward the floor.

6. When you feel at ease with this movement, remove the book, and with even counts, slowly and deeply inhale and exhale, raising and lowering your abdomen. The upper torso should remain passive, with your chest barely moving.

7. You are now breathing abdominally! Practice until the Abdominal Breath is a natural process for you. Now practice it on your hands and knees, letting your abdomen relax toward the floor as you inhale, and then contracting the muscles upward toward your spine as you exhale. Do not arch your spine as you practice. Keep it parallel to the floor—flat, like a table. Practice four breaths in this position. Once you have mastered doing it alone at home, begin to practice at quiet times during the day—at a stop light, while the computer warms up, at the beginning of a meeting. It takes no extra time to change breathing patterns. Breathe abdominally as you drive to work. Breathe abdominally when you are in a line, or waiting on the telephone, and just as you go to sleep. You will be pleased with its effects.

8. Periodically check your breathing and shift to Abdominal Breath if you are not doing so. If it is still difficult to do correctly, repeat the process on your hands and knees or with the book.

Breathe abdominally whenever you are in a stressful situation. The conscious act of abdominal breathing will help you relax as you respond to a situation.

─────── *THE COMPLETE BREATH* ───────

The Complete Breath is emotionally calming and physically energizing. With the Complete Breath one takes in approximately *ten times more air* than with normal unconscious breathing. It increases lung capacity and clears the air passages. The Complete Breath consists of filling the lungs from bottom to top and then completely exhaling all of the air. You learned how to fill the lower part of your lungs in the Abdominal Breath.

1. To clarify what muscles you are using for the Complete Breath, begin in a standing position, and, using your hands, experience the muscle movement in filling the lower, middle, and upper lungs.

   a. Place your hands on your navel and push the abdomen out and in as you did in the Abdominal Breath.

   b. The second set of muscles you use are the intercostal muscles between the ribs. Place the "heel" of your hands (lower palm near your wrist) on each side at your ribs just above your waist. Push in with the heels of your hands, allowing the finger tips to come close together in front. Now take a quick inhalation and see if the fingers separate. Practice several times, squeezing in with your hands on the exhale. Imagine that your hands are a vice constricting your ribs; inhale to break out of the vice, making the distance between the hands widen.

   c. The third set of muscles are in your upper chest and neck. Place one hand on your chest, just below your throat. Inhale fully. Feel your upper chest expand against your hand, and your lower throat muscles contract slightly. In this part of the breath, you are filling the upper portion of your lungs. Do not hunch your shoulders or cave in at your chest. Keep your spine upright in good posture. Fill your upper chest and back. Do it once on the floor, and see if you can feel your upper back push slightly into the floor as your breath fills your upper lungs.

2. To practice the Complete Breath, stretch out on your back.

3. Breathe through your nose.

4. Place one hand on your navel and the other at your ribs.

5. As you inhale, first relax the abdominal muscles and fill the lower lungs, feeling the hand over the navel rising slightly. Second, continue inhaling the same breath, filling the middle portion of your lungs, and feeling the hand at your ribs being pushed out. Third, move one hand to the upper chest and continue inhaling on the same breath, feeling the upper chest rise and upper back expand.

6. As you exhale through your nose, relax the neck muscles and smoothly contract the ribs and abdominal muscles completely, squeezing out the stale air.

7. Repeat again using your hands to feel the expansion. Now do it without the hands. When you inhale, imagine you are filling a large balloon from the bottom to the top.

8. Now practice the Complete Breath standing, and then sitting upright. Be conscious of your posture.

9. Bring your mind into the exercise to deepen the relaxing effects. Experiment with letting an image, color, or word enhance the process. For example, imagine inhaling calmness and peace, and exhaling tension. Inhale crystal blue clear air (calmness), exhale a thick dark cloud (tension). Or keep both inhalation and exhalation on a calming note. For example, inhale the soothing, cooling color of green, and exhale, allowing the calming green to flood your body and mind. Use this image or one of your choice that relaxes you. If you are depressed, you might choose to inhale a vibrant yellow or orange, or inhale a quality such as courage.

10. Once you are comfortable with the Complete Breath, I recommend that you use it on a regular basis every day. When you have mastered it, do a set of three complete breaths five times a day for a week and enjoy the noticeable effects. Do it consciously, with the eyes closed if possible, and the body relaxed. To help you remember to practice, link it to current daily activities. For example, take one or two Complete Breaths after each phone call, just before you eat, before you get out of your car, and when you go to bed.

——— THREE-PART RHYTHMIC BREATH ———

This breathing technique is helpful for all stress symptoms. It reduces restlessness and gives a quiet boost of energy. The Three-Part Rhythmic Breath consists of a Complete Breath inhalation, holding the breath, and then a Complete Breath exhalation. The inhale, hold, and exhale are all to the same count. The following is to a count of six.

1. Practice this technique lying down, sitting, and then standing. Practice all three of the following steps in each position.

2. Inhale a Complete Breath for a count of 6, filling lower lungs to upper chest as described above.

3. Hold your breath for a count of 6.

4. Exhale for a count of 6.

This is a deeply calming exercise, especially if you do it for a full ten rounds. Use it before an important meeting, after your lunch break, and just as you go to sleep.

You may prefer to keep it simple and stay attentive to the physical experience of breathing, or you can add imagery if it helps you relax more deeply. For example, as you inhale you can picture the waves of an ocean gracefully sweeping in, gathering up your tensions and problems as you hold, and sweeping them away as you exhale.

—————— *THE DOUBLE BREATH* ——————

The Double Breath technique is energizing rather than calming, and is therefore most beneficial if you are depressed, bored, feeling fatigued, or lacking in energy. It has a stimulating and invigorating effect, and is excellent for removing residual tension in the body.

1. Practice the Double Breath in a standing position.

2. Inhale through the nose and exhale through the mouth.

3. The rhythm of the breath is to "double inhale" short-long, and to "double exhale" short-long. "Double" means two distinct puffs or draws with a momentary pause between. It is similar to the Complete Breath, but rather than a smooth inhaling and exhaling, inhale quickly and shortly into your slightly relaxed abdominal area, followed by a split-second pause, then continue the *same* inhalation into the ribs and upper chest. In the first phase of the inhalation count one; in the second phase count to four.

4. Exhale in the same rhythm—a short, quick exhale from the upper chest, a quick pause, then continue exhaling on the *same* breath by squeezing the ribs and abdominal muscles, taking four times as long as the first, quick part of the exhalation.

5. Be conscious of the expansion and contraction of the muscles involved in the movement.

6. Do no more than three Double Breaths in a row or you may become dizzy from over-oxygenation.

7. Now tense your muscles progressively from your feet up to your scalp, and then relax the muscles in reverse order, from your head to your feet. This helps release tension in the body.

8. Once you are comfortable tensing and relaxing your body from head-to-toe, add this to the Double Breath. As you do the second part of the inhalation, tense from your feet to your head.

9. As you do the second part of the exhalation, relax from your head to your toes.

10. Practice a set of three Double Breaths, tensing and relaxing as you breathe.

Do this breath whenever you need a quick boost of energy. Long distance runners often use a form of the Double Breath (without the tensing and relaxing) to maximize oxygen intake.

——— Using Conscious Breathing at Work ———

All of my students and clients talk in glowing terms of the impact of these simple but powerful breathing techniques. They take no time at all to do, and regular use gives tremendous benefits. Stress response symptoms seem to magically disappear when you breath consciously. As one client exclaimed, "My friends still recognize me, but I feel like a new person."

The following exercise will help you become more proficient in your practice. Apply the breathing skills you have learned to your daily work routines. In column one, think of work situations in which you might use conscious breathing to calm or energize you. You might want to refer back to your Stress Profile completed in Part I. In the second column, list your stress symptoms, physical, emotional, and behavioral. In the third column, select a breathing technique that works for you from the preceding exercises. Choose the techniques you feel most comfortable with and able to use at work. Below are examples to guide you.

Your Work Stressor	*Your Stress Symptoms*	*Conscious Breathing Technique*
Waiting on the phone	Holding breath, getting impatient	(3) Abdominal Breaths
Important meeting; making a presentation	Tense, stomach in knots, thinking "I'm not prepared for this"	(3) Three-Part Rhythmic Breaths. Imagine inhaling and holding confidence; exhaling worry
Late afternoon, boss hands you a rush project	Fatigue, backache, irritated with boss, feeling overloaded	(3) Double-Breaths followed by (3) Complete Breaths

Your Work Stressor	*Your Stress Symptoms*	*Conscious Breathing Technique*
_____	_____	_____
_____	_____	_____
_____	_____	_____
_____	_____	_____
_____	_____	_____
_____	_____	_____
_____	_____	_____

The following chapters build on the breath. You will be asked to apply conscious deep breathing as you do other exercises. Remember to breathe! In the next chapter you will learn to relax muscles at will, and how to affect your circulatory system. By quieting the breath, relaxing the muscles, and increasing circulation to the hands, you are bringing your physiological responses to stress more under your control.

12

Deep Relaxation

We must slow down enough for nature and for life itself to lend richness and meaning to our lives.

—Angela P. Trafford, *The Heroic Path*

Deep Relaxation is a core technique of stress management. It is an excellent antidote to all types of stress symptoms. One of the most well known forms of Deep Relaxation is Edmond Jacobson's Progressive Muscle Relaxation (PMR) (Jacobson, 1938). Jacobson, a pioneer in relaxation research, developed PMR to treat patients with anxiety. He successfully replaced the use of tranquilizer drugs with instructions on how to avoid inappropriate muscle tension under all conditions. PMR consists of contracting and relaxing major muscle groups. This procedure, in its initial version, consists of approximately fifty one-hour sessions of relaxation training. In each session the patient lies on his back, eyes closed. After three minutes of relaxing muscles, he tenses and relaxes a specific muscle group three times. The whole rest of the hour he goes limp, letting the whole body relax. There is no suggestivity or autosuggestion included. Over time the entire procedure is shortened.

Variations and shortened versions have been developed, and therapists have refined the technique to meet specific therapeutic demands. It is now widely taught by therapists to train people how to relax muscle tension and reduce anxiety and stress (O'Hara, 1990).

The following two techniques, Active and Passive Deep Relaxation, are based on PMR. The other exercises in this chapter expand upon active and passive relaxation by adding visualization, music, or affirmation. The goal of all the exercises is to elicit the relaxation response. After each exercise you will be asked to observe your body. What you will be looking for is relaxed muscles, abdominal breathing, and a quieted mind.

Initially you will practice these techniques lying on the floor in a quiet place with your eyes closed and the lights dim. After you become comfortable with the techniques, you can use them at work, even sitting at your desk in a noisy office. At the end of the chapter, there will be further suggestions and examples of how and when to apply these techniques to deal with your stress response at work.

Deep Relaxation Techniques

——— *Active Deep Relaxation* ———

Find a quiet setting, dim the lights, and stretch out on the floor with your feet shoulder width apart and your arms about one foot away from your body, palms up. If you have a weak, tense, or painful lower back, place a pillow behind your thighs or rest your calves on the seat of a chair. This position slightly extends the lower back, releasing pressure.

To ensure comfort, gently tighten the abdominal muscles and buttocks, pushing the waist towards the floor, and then release. Gently tense the neck and tuck the chin and release. Pull the shoulders away from the ears and towards your feet, then tense and release. Close your eyes and begin to relax and become attentive to the present moment by paying attention to your breathing. Let your breath take its natural rhythm. Become aware of your body, seeking out areas of tension or tightness. Make any adjustments you need to be comfortable.

Focus your attention on each body part as indicated, and gradually tense, relax, and then observe the area. To "tense" an area, contract the muscles, gradually increasing intensity to a full squeeze. The tensing allows you to then actively relax the muscles to a deeper "at rest" level. To "observe" is to notice the difference between the tensed and relaxed muscles. To "observe" also is to experience the sensations in the newly relaxed area. Active Deep Relaxation should take ten minutes to complete. In order to achieve deeper relaxation, you can record the following instructions, and then play the tape for each relaxation session.

- Take three of the short-long Double Breaths, tensing the whole body on the double inhale, relaxing the body as you exhale.

- Point the toes and *tense/relax/observe* the feet.

- Flex the heels (push the heels away from you) and *tense/relax/observe* the legs.

- *Tense/relax/observe* the thighs by pressing down on your heels.

- Curl your toes downward and *tense/relax/observe* the calves.

- Curl your toes toward your head, extending the heels and *tense/relax/observe* the shins.

- *Tense/relax/observe* the buttocks.

- *Tense/relax/observe* the abdominal area.

- Relax the whole lower body, feeling it relax.

- Now focus on your upper body.

- Press the shoulder blades into the floor, raising the chest slightly, and *tense/relax/observe* the shoulder blades and chest.

- Curl the shoulders toward the ceiling and tuck the chin, and *tense/relax/observe* the upper back.

- Make the hands into fists and *tense/relax/observe* the hands.

- Flex wrists toward ceiling and *tense/relax/observe* the lower arms and hands.

- Flex wrists toward floor and *tense/relax/observe* the upper arms and hands.

- Shrug shoulders and *tense/relax/observe* shoulders.

- Press head against floor and *tense/relax/observe* neck.

- Purse lips, tense throat, then open mouth wide, relax the tongue, lower jaw, and lips.

- Scrunch face, knit eyebrows, *relax/observe* face.

- Pause for three natural breaths, then focus on the entire body.

- Scan the body for any tension and *tense/relax/observe* any area still holding tension. Keep letting go deeper and deeper.

- Take six slow Abdominal Breaths, smoothly relaxing your abdominal muscles as you inhale and gently contracting them as you exhale, relaxing more deeply with each exhalation.

- Gently wiggle the fingers and toes.

- Rock the head gently from side to side.

- Bend the knees into the chest and clasp your hands around your shins and gently rock from side to side several times.

- Slowly come up into a sitting position.

If you have done the exercise correctly, you will now experience the relaxation response. Observe your body. Are you breathing abdominally? Are your muscles relaxed? Are your hands warm? These are physiological indications telling you that you have successfully elicited the relaxation response. These indications are the biological feedback evidenced when you are truly relaxed.

With your eyes still closed, experience how it feels to have your muscles relaxed and yet filled with energy. Enjoy a minute of peace and tranquility. You might use the time to repeat an affirmation, such as: "Harmony and peace now fill my being." Open your eyes and observe the quiet of the room around you. Then begin your activities (O'Hara, 1990).

Active Deep Relaxation adapts beautifully to on-site practice. Once you have enjoyed and mastered the technique, begin to do mini-versions of it at work. While at your work area, pause, take a Complete Breath and then tense and relax three times in areas where you are holding tension. For example, take a deep breath and then tense and relax your shoulders three times. Repeat the process for your neck and upper back.

——— PASSIVE DEEP RELAXATION ———

In the first phase of Passive Deep Relaxation you focus your attention on each body part to become aware of the sensations and possible tension in the particular body part, and then release the tension by consciously relaxing the area. You do not actively tense each body part separately before relaxing it as in Active Deep Relaxation. Instead, there are just a few general tensing and relaxing actions. Take approximately five minutes for this phase. In Phase Two you will learn relaxing visualizations to deepen your relaxation response. I recommend that you make a tape of these instructions for your relaxation sessions.

Phase One: The Body

Stretch out on your back. Extend your legs or rest your calves on a chair. Place your palms upward, a foot or so away from your body. Close your eyes. Take a Complete Breath, entirely filling your lungs and then exhaling completely. Take a second Complete Breath, tensing gently from toes to head on the inhalation and consciously relaxing from head to toes on the exhalation. Take a third Complete Breath, lifting your head, arms, and legs several inches off the floor while tensing the whole body as hard as you can on the inhalation, and releasing the head, arms, and legs down to the floor on the exhalation. Push the small of your back into the floor while tensing the buttocks and the abdominal muscles.

Next push the shoulder blades into the floor and lift the chest slightly. At the same time push the back of your neck gently toward the floor, tucking the chin and pulling the shoulders towards your feet.

Relax and make any adjustments you need to be comfortable. Now you will use the power of your focused attention to consciously relax every cell in your body.

- Bring your attention down into your feet and become aware of how they feel. Consciously relax them.

- Now be attentive to the shins and calves. Become aware of and experience this part of your body. Consciously let go of any residual tension there.

- Focus your mind on the thighs and be aware of the sensations there; then release more deeply.

- Observe the abdominal area and then soften there.

- Continue observing, experiencing, and relaxing each body part:

  Observe/experience/relax the buttocks.

  Observe/experience/relax the rib cage area.

  Observe/experience/relax the upper chest and upper back.

  Observe/experience/relax the shoulders.

  Observe/experience/relax the upper arms.

  Observe/experience/relax the lower arms.

  Observe/experience/relax the hands.

  Observe/experience/relax the neck and throat.

  Observe/experience/relax the tongue and inside the mouth.

  Observe/experience/relax each part of the face.

  Observe/experience/relax the scalp.

As you did after the first relaxation exercise, observe your body. Are you breathing abdominally? Are your muscles relaxed? Are your hands warm? If so, you are truly relaxed.

Phase Two: The Mind

Now that your body is deeply relaxed, continue to keep your eyes closed and use the next five minutes to quiet your mind. Use one of the following methods.

Relax with Music. Have soft music playing during Passive Deep Relaxation Phase One. After relaxing the body parts, focus on the music. If your mind wanders from the present moment, gently bring it back into the sound of the music. Anchor your mind to the present with the music. Do not *try* to listen, *allow* yourself to listen. Let it flow through you. Trying or willing the mind into the present can raise your blood pressure. Instead, observe when your mind has wandered, and, without guilt or disappointment in yourself, bring your attention back to the sound. Listen to the notes, the sounds, and the pauses without analyzing them. Use music that is peaceful and calming. Choose music that soothes you and helps you to focus on the present experience. Avoid music that girds you to action or reminds you of the past.

Discard Pain. Scan the body for tension; relax wherever you find it. If you have an area that is chronically sore, focus your attention there and take a minute to experience the sensations there. Mentally document the tingling, pressure, warmth, or other sensations you are feeling. You will notice that pain lessens by as much as half by discarding the label "pain," and without judgment or avoidance, observe with detachment the sensations of the traumatized area. Like a scientist gathering data, objectively note what the body is experiencing in the area. As a final step, think of a color that appeals to you at the moment, and imagine the area filling with the color. It may be easier to imagine if you *breathe* a color into the area.

Inspirational Relaxers. Choose an affirmation, scriptural passage, poem, or inspiring quotation and repeat it to yourself or have it recorded on a tape. An affirmation I enjoy is, "Amidst life's storms I stand serene." Another uplifting image is, "My boat of life floats lightly on tides of peace" (Kriyananda, 1991).

Complete Phase Two by taking a Complete Breath, fully filling the lungs as you inhale. Gently wiggle your fingers and toes. Bring your knees to your chest, rock side to side, then come into a sitting position. With eyes still closed, observe the effects of consciously relaxing. Next open your eyes and take a minute to be still, remaining in the quiet attitude of the relaxation exercise (O'Hara, 1990).

Visualization

Visualization is a powerful tool for replacing negative images and thoughts with positive ones. Your stress is reduced by taking a mental break from your problems. By using all of your senses in the imagery, your body responds to your calming imaginary scene by relaxing.

When people are stressed, they visualize pressing scenarios. The overdue paperwork, the impending decisions, the conflict with a supervisor all crowd the mind with worry thoughts or a sense of overwhelm. The mental input from the cortex of the brain goes to the limbic system (emotional brain). The visualization of disaster heightens emotions which are translated through the limbic-hypothalamus-pituitary axis into an outpouring of adrenaline, accelerated heartbeat, shallow breathing, increased blood pressure, and other physiological stress responses. As explained more fully in Chapter 3, the limbic system is unable to differentiate between visualization of catastrophe and reality. Just as thoughts of eating a favorite food causes the mouth to water, anxious thoughts cause corresponding physiological responses.

Visualization is therefore an important—and enjoyable—tool in stress management. After consciously slowing your breath, relaxing your body, and quieting your emotions, you will visualize that you are in a safe, calm, enjoyable setting. Your limbic-hypothalamus-pituitary axis acts as if you *are* in that reality. Physiological responses might include reduced blood pressure, reduced heart rate, and other bodily relaxation responses.

——— Deep Relaxation with Visualization ———

Phase One: The Body

Dim the lights and stretch out on your back, using a pillow under your thighs if needed. Close your eyes. Take three short-long Double Breaths, tensing and relaxing with each breath. Follow with three Complete Breaths, filling the lungs entirely and remembering to concentrate on your body and the flow of air. Now let the breath take its natural rhythm.

Relax your body from your feet to your head, focusing on each body part and consciously letting go as you did in Passive Deep Relaxation. Take approximately five minutes to relax the whole body. It is helpful to imagine breathing space and relaxation into each area. Once you are relaxed, begin the following visualization. Again, you might record this to help you relax more fully. Spend about five minutes visualizing.

Phase Two: Visualization

Imagine yourself on an empty beach of white sand . . . Vibrant green palm trees gently sway in the background . . . Feel the warmth of the sand beneath you. Allow yourself to sink deeper into its white softness as it contours to your relaxing muscles. Let sand sift through your fingers . . . Feel the rays of the sun warming and penetrating your palms and fingers and thumbs . . . Feel the tingling warm sensation in your hands. Now feel the warmth of the sun on your feet, penetrating the skin, warming the muscles and tissues.

Now feel the cool soft breeze blow across your face and through your hair . . . Let the wind remove your lingering thoughts. Your mind is now cool, quiet, empty. Feel the cool breeze entering the brain . . . Smell the fragrance of the sea . . . See the deep blue ocean with sunlight dancing on the surface, and the roll of gentle waves breaking on the shore . . . Let the sound cascade over you. Observe the crystal blue of the sky . . . a bird soaring high above . . . you are cleansed and nurtured by the natural beauty around you . . . you are open to its healing presence . . .

Feel yourself sink deeper into the softness of the sand, muscles relaxing, deeper and deeper. Feel the weight of your body as you let go more deeply . . . Feel yourself light as a feather, your mind unburdened. Let your consciousness lift and soar. Be free! . . . Become aware now of being on the floor, your mind quiet and body relaxed. Take two Complete Breaths and stretch or do what feels comfortable for you; open your eyes when you are ready. Come up into a sitting position. Take three Double Breaths and step back into your day, relaxed and refreshed from your mini-vacation!

Themes for visualization can be personalized. Visualize your favorite place in nature and experience the colors and shapes. Note the sky of your special place. Perhaps you see the sky through a canopy of spreading, leafy oak tree branches, or your sky has fluffy clouds or a wispy rainbow. Perhaps you lie on a cushion of velvety soft moss, or you feel the cooling waters of a stream as you immerse yourself into the cleansing waters. Wherever your journey takes you, let each of your senses experience your favorite place and then open yourself to the beauty around you, feeling, perhaps, a kinship with all life.

You may want to personalize a visualization by seeing the details of a favorite past occasion or a projected blissful future event. Or drop off your day pack of worries and take a magical journey!

Deep Relaxation and Specific Stress Responses

The object of all the relaxation techniques is two-fold: first, to experience the benefit of quieting your body through the techniques, and second, eventually to use the techniques during a stress response.

Insomnia

Is it difficult for you to go to sleep? Do you wake up and then toss and turn at 4 a.m., unable to go back to sleep? If you are experiencing insomnia, use the Deep Relaxation with Visualization. Many, many of my clients have used it with great success. Having consciously relaxed mentally and physically, your sleep will be deeper and you will feel more refreshed in the morning.

Anxiety

Other clients have found real benefit doing Deep Relaxation in the midst of a hectic day. One teacher closes her classroom door and takes a restoring ten-minute relaxation break rather than going to the noisy, crowded faculty lounge. A secretary does a relaxation at the beginning of her lunch break. A government employee has found refuge in his car for deep relaxation. A woman who does data entry all day "regains her sanity" with a three-minute stretching routine followed by breathing, relaxation, and visualization at her terminal each mid-morning and afternoon. One manager tells his secretary, "I cannot be disturbed due to an important engagement."

With management's support, relaxation breaks can become an integral part of the work day. At a distributing company in northern California and a national database marketing firm north of Sacramento, employees and management get together to stretch and do Deep Relaxation as a group.

Gradually you will master the techniques and be able to respond to stress with conscious calm breathing, relaxed muscles, and warm hands. Some people visualize themselves in a bubble of calm, with the stressor outside of its shielding perimeter.

Migraine Headaches

A migraine headache is often a symptom of stress. Practice each of the above relaxation skills until they are second nature to you. The ability to elicit the relaxation response through Abdominal Breath, muscle relaxation, and quieting the mind is an important part of headache control. Remember, do not *try* to relax; rather, *allow* yourself to let go. In addition, don't analyze your current stressful situation while you have a migraine.

Stress can cause a change in blood flow, which can result in a migraine headache. Do you tend to have cold clammy hands or feet when you are stressed? When under pressure the sympathetic nervous system causes our peripheral blood vessels to constrict, resulting in cold hands and feet. At the same time, the head heats up due to the increased flow of blood to the head. To combat a migraine headache, use a visualization which reverses the temperatures. Once you have relaxed, visualize less flow of blood to the brain and more flow to the hands, or create your own visualization which should include warming the hands and cooling the head. The purpose is to constrict the blood vessels in the brain and open the peripheral capillaries in your hands and feet. You can use the previous visualization of lying on the beach; the key elements in that visualization are the focus on cooling the head and warming the hands and feet.

An additional feature which helps many people is to end the visualization with a sensation of feeling heavy and then feeling light. Feeling heavy is related to the increase of blood into the relaxed area due to the opening of the capillaries. The sensation of lightness follows as you release the burden of worries. In the previous visualization, I have included this concept, using the sensation of first sinking deeper into the sand and then floating like a feather.

In addition, before doing the visualization, it can be helpful to warm your hands by briefly soaking them in warm water, and then placing a cool damp cloth on your forehead as you do the visualization.

As you continue to practice, your ability to elicit the relaxation response will improve. One client experienced severe migraines. She would lose her peripheral vision, then experience jagged, rainbow-colored lightning flashes. The migraine mushroomed into a pounding four-hour headache. By lying down, consciously relaxing and visualizing, she eliminated the pounding headache. With further practice she shortened the rainbow lightning phase. In time she could stop the loss of peripheral vision and prevent the whole process. At one session she proudly announced she was able to short-circuit all phases during a business meeting without anyone being aware of what she was doing.

USING DEEP RELAXATION AT WORK

The following is a quick-relax version of Active Deep Relaxation. Once you have mastered the technique in a quiet setting, you can use this method to achieve muscle relaxation quickly. You can successfully use this abbreviated version to release muscular tension at work. When tensing muscles, gradually contract muscles from low to medium to high tension. Do not excessively tense the muscles, as it can cause muscle cramping. Take five to ten seconds to tighten muscles. Hold for 5 seconds, and then take 20-30 seconds to relax. Practice standing or sitting.

1. Take one Complete Breath, filling the lungs completely as you inhale, and consciously relaxing as you exhale.

2. Scrunch face, push neck back slightly and tense, lift and tense shoulders. Hold. Relax.

3. Curl hands into fists, tighten lower arms, then biceps and chest. Hold. Relax.

4. Tense buttocks, abdomen, and stomach. Hold. Relax.

5. Curl toes, tense calves and thighs. Hold. Relax.

6. Inhale, tensing muscles in a wave from toes to head. Exhale, relaxing muscles in a wave from head to toes.

Personalized Version

1. Take one Complete Breath, as above.

2. Tense, hold, and relax in any area you feel tension. For example, curl shoulders and tense, hold, relax.

3. Repeat step two twice.

Now think of a few work situations where you might use Deep Relaxation. Before doing this exercise again, go back over the Stress Profile you filled out in Part I identifying your stressors and symptoms. The following examples provide a guideline.

Your Work Stressors	Your Stress Symptoms	Deep Relaxation Technique
Disagreeable telephone call	Tense shoulders, neck	Quik-relax version while caller talks
Information overload	Headache, fuzzy thinking, confusion	Visualization of favorite nature scene with music at lunch break
Noisy work environment	Irritable, edgy, distracted, tense muscles	Visualization: A tropical breeze cleansing body/mind at desk

Your Work Stressors	*Your Stress Symptoms*	*Deep Relaxation Technique*
_____	_____	_____
_____	_____	_____
_____	_____	_____
_____	_____	_____
_____	_____	_____

You can also elicit the relaxation response through meditation, an outstanding technique in your arsenal of weapons to combat stress. The next chapter instructs you in the art of meditation. It too adapts easily to on-site practice.

13

Meditation

Nourishing our spirit is necessary if we want healthy self-esteem.

—California Task Force to Promote
Self-Esteem

Meditation "takes the edge off" at work.

—William Coors

Meditation has come out of the ashram and into the office. From top management to clerks, workers are using meditation to calm the mind and relieve stress symptoms. People who meditate regularly say it also results in increased productivity, reduced irritability, and improved ability to cope with job pressures (Lowlier, 1993). Many also say it brings increased peace of mind, which in turn brings more joy in their lives and a clearer sense of purpose.

Meditation is a close relative to prayer. In prayer you talk with your heart; in meditation you listen with your heart. Meditation is central to some of the most ancient spiritual traditions in the world, but whether in or out of its spiritual context, meditation is an excellent tool for stress management. Modern scientific studies have confirmed the therapeutic value of meditation to reduce multiple stress symptoms. It successfully elicits the relaxation response for relief of anxiety and a host of other physical and emotional maladies.

The Quiet Mind

The goal of previous chapters focused primarily on physical relaxation. The aim of meditation is to achieve a deeper mental quieting by silencing our constantly repeated mental tapes and aimless mental chatter. Meditation is the most beneficial of all exercises for relieving mental and emotional stress. One cannot continue at a faster and faster pace and remain healthy. A mental time-out for a minimum of ten minutes daily restores the balance of *being* with the *doing* in life. These mental mini-vacations for letting go of worries and pressures return one to a sense of wholeness.

Meditation is the repeated practice of attempting to keep the attention on one designated object, thought, or image. The meditator repeatedly refocuses on the object of concentration without judging or criticizing the busy mind for wandering. Training the naturally busy mind in one-pointed concentration helps to stop the torrent of thoughts and repeated worrisome images that can be the downfall in stress management.

What if you are unable to stop the nagging, persistent thoughts? Rather than becoming a victim of your thoughts you can use meditation as a tool to gain entrance into your thought process. The practice of meditation teaches you to observe your thought patterns. This knowledge enables you to catch a typical direction or line of thought in its initial stages and replace it with the object of concentration. Or you can learn to replace it with a positive thought. You can stand at the gateway of your mind and with discrimination, choose what thoughts to think. Exercises at the end of this chapter will help you to use meditation to become more aware of your thought processes. Later chapters will provide further instruction on how to replace negative thinking patterns with positive ones.

William Coors, chairman of Adolf Coors Company, has been meditating for years, ten times a week for 20 minutes each session. The Coors Company Wellness Program combines meditation, nutrition, and exercise to control health care costs. The program has been extremely successful, a major factor in lowering the company's mental health costs 27 percent between 1987 and 1993 (Lowlier, 1993).

The Mind/Body Medical Institute at Harvard University produced such a wealth of research information on the success of meditation in reducing stress that twelve Boston-area employers, including Polaroid and Marriott, have participated in the Institute's corporate program of yoga, meditation, and guided visual imagery (Benson, 1976). Dr. Herbert Benson, founder of the Institute, has done extensive research for over 25 years on the benefits of eliciting the relaxation response, particularly through meditation. According to Dr. Benson, the four prerequisites to eliciting the relaxation response through meditation are:

1. a quiet environment

2. a comfortable sitting position

3. a mental device such as a word or a phase repeated over and over to break stressful thinking patterns

4. an attitude that permits the relaxation to happen at its own pace, without force and without guilt feelings if your mind wanders

Incorporating these four elements into a ten to twenty minute meditation once or twice a day will markedly enhance your well-being (Benson, 1976).

Note: Do not meditate if you are clinically depressed or experiencing any psychotic or hallucinatory symptoms. Instead, take a walk in a pleasant setting, do some of the office exercises, or seek support from a friend or counselor.

——— *HOW TO MEDITATE* ———

Choose a quiet setting. Sit in a straight-backed chair. If you have lower back problems which interfere with your concentration, use a pillow behind your lower back, or meditate while lying on your back, with your calves resting on a chair or pillow. Do what is necessary to be comfortable. It is best to sit because when you lie down the tendency is to fall asleep.

Close your eyes and practice the Double Breath three times, including the tensing and relaxing. Follow with a series of three Three-Part Rhythmic Breaths. They will help you begin the quieting process and bring your attention into the present moment.

Let your breath take its natural rhythm. Without interfering with your breath or trying to control it, repeat a word, phrase, or short prayer. Repeat the word on both inhalation and exhalation. For example, inhale silently saying "relaxing"; exhale, again silently saying "relaxing." If you are using a longer phrase, repeat the first half of the phrase during inhalation, and the second half during exhalation. You could inhale, silently repeating "I am," and exhale, silently repeating "letting go."

Two keys: first, always allow the breath to follow its natural rhythm. Second, if your mind wanders, bring it back to the anchor of the breath and the phrase *without self-condemnation*. Initially your mind may *appear* more active than before meditation, but that is only because of your increased awareness of your thoughts. With practice, your mind will quiet.

After practicing for ten minutes, let go of the focus on the breath and the word or phrase and enjoy the inner quiet and peace for a few minutes. When you are ready, open your eyes, and sit quietly. To refocus on your outer environment, take several Double Breaths and stretch before getting up from the chair.

To help incorporate meditation into your daily routine, meditate at a specific time each day. The best way to make it a habit is to meditate at a designated time and place. You can always *add* spontaneous times!

Meditation is one of the most powerful techniques at your disposal. Follow the above format and then personalize it to meet your needs and spiritual inclinations. For example, after focusing on the breath and the phrase, finish your meditation with several minutes of enjoying the peace, praying, resolving a personal issue, or doing whatever feels appropriate to you.

———— *USING MEDITATION AT WORK* ————

Go over your work day to discover when and where you can meditate regularly. Can you squeeze in a ten-minute meditation at lunch or just before everyone else arrives? Can you meditate in your car, at a nearby park, or in a quiet spot in your building? Meditating with someone else may make it easier to find a place to meditate and is a good support for keeping up the practice. Fill out the following.

When can I meditate at work? _____

Where can I meditate at work? _____

Is there someone I can meditate with? _____

What word or phrase will I repeat? _____

Other Forms of Meditation

Quiet Time

Quiet Time is an excellent adaptation of meditation. Quiet Time is attention in the present moment, whether being physically active or inactive. A solitary walk while attentive to sensations, gardening with your mind in the activity, or hiking while observing the beauty around you are all calming. Quiet Time also includes reading, doing crossword puzzles, or watching the sun set. The best Wellness Program includes times of quiet and times of enjoyment. They can be spontaneous, frivolous, organized, with others or alone. The trick is to be "in the present" and not to worry. This is the challenge!

Every hectic schedule needs to be balanced with relaxation and enjoyment. My clients have found Quiet Time solutions in comedy movies, inspirational reading, camping, star gazing, rock climbing, and stamp collecting. How do you need to re-balance your scales? You have options!

Creative Time

Creative Time is another excellent adaptation of meditation. Have you dropped pleasurable hobbies or activities due to lack of time? Have you stopped expressing yourself through writing or art? These are wonderful outlets for releasing pent-up emotions and worries. You can create the time for these activities if you make up your mind to do so. Look at your schedule and find a regular, brief if necessary, space for these activities. This type of time-out re-energizes you and clears your mind for better solutions to the challenges in your life. It also makes you more pleasant to be around!

——— USING CREATIVE/QUIET TIME AT WORK ———

Use the space below to list Quiet Time or Creative Time substitutes for regular meditation practice at work. For example, bring a good novel to read at lunch or your embroidery work.

1. _____

2. _____

3. _____

4. _____

Journaling

One particularly helpful form of Creative Time for stress management is journaling. Write out your feelings and perceptions as they come to you. Buy yourself a journal or notebook to write in before or after work or on your breaks.

Journaling gives you the opportunity to clarify what is bothering you, so that you can look at healthier solutions. At times it is helpful to journal in letter form. You may want to express your feelings to your supervisor in this format. The purpose is not to send the letter, but to write and rewrite the letter to release your feelings and reduce the intensity of your pain. As you rewrite, you find the emotions become less intense or change in focus. It's an excellent way to sort out your feelings.

You can use the following format when making your work-related entries.

1. Describe your work stressor(s) (interpersonal or situational).

2. Write out your feelings and perceptions, in the form of a letter if helpful.

3. List possible healthy options to resolve the stressor(s) or relieve your distress.

An additional step you can take is to go back over what you wrote and look for thinking patterns. Also when you were meditating, did you notice any repeated thoughts? Use both meditation practice and journaling to become more aware of the progression of your thoughts when your mind wanders from its designated focus.

For example, when a client of mine read over his afternoon journal entry, he noticed his thoughts at one point became very pessimistic.

He'd written: "I'm overwhelmed with all my work projects. I'll never get them done in time. I might as well give up now. I was never any good at this type of work anyway."

The purpose of meditation is not to stop such thoughts but to observe them, let them go, and return to your one focus. However, in Chapter 18, you will have an opportunity to examine your thoughts more closely in order to gain more control and direct them in healthier, less stressful progressions. Then you can rewrite your thoughts.

> *The client above rewrote: "I'm overwhelmed with all my work. I can take it a step at a time. I can delegate and prioritize. I have the ability to do the job."*

If you find, after practicing the techniques of Conscious Breathing, Deep Relaxation, and Meditation, that you are still having difficulty achieving the relaxation response, the following chapter may help you.

14

The Phenomenon of Biofeedback

We can counter the pervasiveness of stress with techniques which promote deep relaxation.

—Judith Green, *Biofeedback Training*

Biofeedback can be amazingly effective in gaining self-regulation of internal states. Any physiological process that you can continuously monitor you can bring under a degree of conscious control (Norris, 1986). Even so-called involuntary systems (not under our conscious control) such as the nervous system, stomach, heart, and intestines can be controlled and will respond to volition and visualization (Norris, 1986). If you have been unable to elicit the relaxation response, biofeedback can be very helpful. You will need to go to a counselor trained in biofeedback to use this technique.

Biofeedback uses instruments to monitor your body to help you teach yourself how to gain control of a wide variety of internal physiological activities. These instruments inform you of the effects of your mind on your body, and what you need to do to change or slow down a physiological response. Through lights, beeping sounds, or other indicators you can watch your thoughts or emotions speed up your heart or increase your blood pressure or respiration. Alternately, these instruments show you how meditation or visualization slows down those internal systems and produces a relaxation response by providing information on whether you have lowered your body temperature, relaxed your muscles, or slowed your heart rate.

Biofeedback and Conscious Control

In 1970 Swami Rama, an Indian adept, agreed to be tested for five weeks at the Menninger Clinic's Center for Applied Psychophysiology. In one experiment he deliberately stopped his heart by putting it into atrial fibrillation for 17 seconds. In another experiment he controlled vascular behavior in his hand so that two areas of his right palm, 2 inches apart, were made to differ by 10 degrees Fahrenheit as measured by thermistors attached to his palm. The experiment lasted 20 minutes, with his hands remaining in an open, palms-up, relaxed position (Norris, 1989b). Swami Rama stated that this was one of the most difficult psychophysical controls he had learned.

Swami Rama's ability to control physiological functions with his mind is remarkable. Equally impressive, however, is that a graduate student at the clinic taught himself to accomplish the same voluntary control of blood flow to the two locations on his palms in one week! The student used a biofeedback machine informing him of skin temperature changes as slight as 1/100 degree Fahrenheit (Norris, 1989b).

These two men are striking examples of the phenomenon of body/mind connection. Much of stress management is based on the growing body of scientific information that our thoughts and emotions directly affect our bodies, including our immune system.

The underlying premise for teaching relaxation skills and how to change thoughts and attitudes into a more positive framework is that these skills not only help you feel more relaxed and happy, they directly affect your physical health.

Using Biofeedback to Reduce Work Stress

Biofeedback is a tool to enhance self-regulation for all clients with many illnesses, not only those whose illness is related to stress. But because stress exacerbates any disease and inhibits the immune system, a basic starting point with arrivals at the Menninger Clinic Center for Applied Psychophysiology is to teach them how to relax. The Center regularly observes an immediate change in the patient through the simple technique of Deep Relaxation taught with the help of biofeedback instruments (telephone interview with Nina Meyer, The Menninger Clinic, 17 September, 1993).

Biofeedback is a remarkable tool for gaining conscious control of biological systems. If you have been unable to elicit the relaxation response, or want to fine-tune self-regulation of a specific physiological system, I recommend you investigate its use.

If you think biofeedback may be helpful, look for a therapist who is trained in biofeedback. Such a person may be available through your Employee Assistance Program (EAP). See Chapters 24 and 25 for more information regarding employee mental health benefits. Whether through your EAP or your medical insurance, call and ask for information regarding your outpatient mental health benefits. Request a counselor who is trained in biofeedback for relaxation therapy.

15

Physical Activities for Stress Reduction and Wellness

Unhappy business men, I am convinced, would increase their happiness more by walking six miles every day than by any conceivable change of philosophy.

—Bertrand Russell

I like long walks, especially when they are taken by people who annoy me.

—Fred Allen

The object of this chapter is to convince you of the many physical and mental benefits of exercise and to give you examples of how to fit it into your busy work schedule. People who work full time, even extra hours, often drop exercise because they don't have time or feel exhausted. "Accumulated" exercise, discussed later in this chapter, is a perfect solution for the employee with no time to spare. Today more and more jobs are of a sedentary nature and in closed, often stuffy, office environments, which use forced air heating and air conditioning.

Lack of physical movement and lack of fresh air cause exhaustion and are major contributors to job stress. Exercise is an excellent means for reducing the effects of these job stressors.

The benefits of physical activity are legendary—one of the greatest being that it reduces depression and anxiety. Ask anyone who is physically active: you *feel* better when you exercise! It alters your mood. People who exercise on a regular basis derive vast psychological benefits.

I have repeatedly found that I am more enthusiastic, think more clearly, feel better about myself, and bring a greater level of inner harmony to everything I do when I exercise regularly and eat moderately. From my own experience, and the experience of thousands of my ice skating, dance, and fitness students as well as my clients, I say, "Do it. You will be thrilled with the process and the results."

Exercise is not only a main ingredient of well-being, it is usually a rather accurate barometer of self-care. Because an overstressed or depressed person is likely to drop exercise, the very activity most needed to turn the mind in a positive direction, I make my clients acutely aware of the strongly mood-altering effects of exercise and help them find forms of exercise that they like.

How Aerobic Activity Alters Negative Moods

The statistics support my exuberance. Repeatedly, studies confirm that exercise will improve your mood and decrease your anxiety and tension. The California Human Performance Laboratories, the Mayo Clinic, Purdue University, the Cooper Clinic, and numerous other research centers have found a direct link between physical health and psychological well-being. People who exercise regularly tend to be more imaginative, self-sufficient, resolute, and emotionally stable. A mere ten minutes of vigorous exercise doubles the body's level of epinephrine, a hormone linked with feelings of euphoria (Boga, 1993). Exercise alone increases self-esteem, improves one's attitude toward work, and increases creativity and concentration (Cooper, 1978).

Anecdotal stories in *Prevention* magazine and elsewhere, including numerous reports by psychotherapists, also validate the impact of exercise and sound nutrition on stress reduction. The more you take charge of your life by exercising and eating nutritiously, the better you will feel physically and mentally. You feel good and you look good when you exercise.

Increasing Longevity Through Physical Activity

Appropriate exercise not only reduces stress but also minimizes the risk of heart attack, increases good (HDL) cholesterol, improves productivity, promotes weight control, tempers back pain, and increases longevity. "Fitness puts more years in your life and more life in your years," says Dr. Kenneth Cooper, founder of the Cooper Institute for Aerobics Research in Dallas (Cooper, 1978).

Dr. Cooper, a leading advocate and expert on physical fitness, states that physical fitness gives you more energy on both a physical and psychological-emotional level. According to a model developed by RAND Corporation, each mile run or walked by a sedentary person increases their life span by 21 minutes (Boga, 1993). Before his death in 1994, George Sheehan, M.D., triathlete and Medical Editor for *Runner's World*, agreed that exercise can greatly reduce our rate of aging, especially if weight is maintained (Boga, 1993).

According to the President's Council on Physical Fitness and Sports, only 20 percent of the public exercises at a level recommended for cardiovascular benefit, and at least 40 percent of the American public are completely sedentary. Back problems, a leading cause of absenteeism and disability in the corporate environment, can be largely attributed to a completely sedentary life style (President's Council, 1993a).

The leading cause of death in the U.S. is heart attack, followed by cancer, strokes, and other blood-vessel diseases. Heart and blood-vessel diseases lead to more deaths than all other causes of death combined. Approximately 70 million Americans have one or more forms of cardiovascular disease, and about 30 percent of U.S. adults have high blood pressure. In the U. S., more than 1.5 million heart attacks occur each year, and someone dies of cardiovascular disease every 34 seconds, or nearly one million people annually (President's Council, 1993c). This accounts for 55 percent of all deaths in the country. One man in three will have symptomatic arterial disease before age 60. Of these cases, 40 percent will have their first and only symptom—death (Cooper, 1978).

A wealth of studies conclusively show that sedentary people are more susceptible to heart disease than active people. For example, one study which followed 16,936 Harvard alumni for 16 years (1962-1978), found that those who exercised regularly had 50 percent fewer deaths from heart disease than those who did not exercise (Boga, 1993).

There is dramatic evidence that aerobic exercise successfully combats heart disease and stroke. Of the eleven factors which affect the probability of getting heart disease (heredity, stress, diet, fat abnormalities, hypertension, heartbeat abnormalities, diabetes, obesity, smoking, age, and lack of physical activity) only your age and your genes will not be changed for the better by running, walking, or some other form of aerobic activity (Boga, 1993). "Aerobic" means exercising at 65 to 80 percent of your "target heart rate." Achieving your target heart rate will be discussed in the next section.

How to Maximize Benefits of Exercise

When you exercise, be sure to take a break from internal pressures too. One reason for the release of stress is the "time-out effect" of exercise. Leave the pressures behind while you work out. There are no phones, no unfinished papers in front of you. Perhaps initially let your mind sort through its worries, but then *consciously* take a mental break. Take a mental time-out—a Worry Break—from worry thoughts. A Worry Break means keeping your attention in the present. Involve your mind in the physical activity or your surroundings. If you have trouble keeping your attention in the present, take a Worry Break by anchoring yourself in the moment by counting "one, two, one, two," keeping rhythm with your activity. Visualize the numbers in your head and count the movements. If your mind wanders, gently and without guilt bring it back to the counting or a chosen phrase as you practiced in the meditation exercise. This Worry Break technique can be used in connection with any activity. It will help you keep focused. It is especially helpful to exercise outside, in a natural setting.

Often a mental break allows you to solve problems because the exercise has lifted you out of a negative mood. Your options are no longer clouded by anxiety or depression.

When exercising for stress reduction, the key is not to become competitive or rigid in your practice. Except for overly competitive athletes for whom the drive for success creates its own stress, the vast majority of people find that physical activity leaves them relaxed yet invigorated. You will derive the same physical benefits and profit more psychologically if you exercise with a noncompetitive attitude and enjoy the experience.

If You Hate to Exercise

One highly stressed patient told me, "I don't do the outdoors or exercise of any kind." She is one of the holdouts who vehemently opposes exercise, or nutritional changes, or refuses or is unable to quit smoking. For these clients particularly, it is important to engage in some of the other techniques of stress management. She ended up reducing her stress through relaxation techniques and improved communication skills. Once she could voice her feelings clearly and without antagonism, her anxiety was greatly reduced.

Although I encourage you to be physically active, if you still feel resistant, just keep the above information as a seed for thought and possible future use. True stress management is shedding your stress using those techniques that feel comfortable to you and appropriate to your situation.

How Intensely and How Often?

How much and how often do you need to exercise to experience wonderful results? There has been a dramatic shift of opinion on the amount and intensity of exercise needed to effect physical and emotional changes.

Heart rate is widely accepted as a good method for measuring intensity during exercise. The heart rate you should maintain is called your "target heart rate." In 1975 the American College of Sports Medicine recommended that the minimum target heart rate during exercise be 80 percent of the heart's maximum capacity. Continued research has found physical and psychological benefits at lower and lower heart rates. In 1980 the goal was 70 percent; in 1986 it was 60 percent; in 1992, the minimum target heart rate dropped to a range of 50 to 60 percent of the heart's maximum capacity (Painton, 1993).

One of the simplest ways to arrive at your target heart rate is as follows. First determine your maximum heart rate, which is 220 minus your age. Multiply this number by the percentage accepted by you or your doctor. For example, if the accepted goal is 60 percent of maximum heart rate, the target heart rate of a 40-year-old would be 60 percent of 220 minus 40, or (220-40) multiplied by .60, or 108.

When checking heart rate during a workout, take your pulse within five seconds after interrupting exercise because it starts to go down once you stop moving. Count your pulse for ten seconds and multiply by six to get the per-minute rate. The above formula for determining your target heart rate applies to about 60 percent of the American population. If you have a fast beating heart, a slow beating heart, or are on cardiovascular medication, the formula is less useful. Determine your personal target heart rate with your physician. *Use common sense*. Be kind and patient with yourself. If you are gasping for air you are overdoing, even if you are walking at a slow pace for a short distance. The Talk Test is an accurate formula for everyone: if you are unable to talk, you are overexerting yourself (Bailey, 1991).

Three American authorities on fitness and health—the U.S. Centers for Disease Control and Prevention, the American College of Sports Medicine, and the President's Council on Physical Fitness and Sports—issued a joint report in July 1993, which formulated a new recommendation regarding the amount of activity needed to prevent disease. After reviewing persuasive scientific evidence gathered over the past several decades, they concluded that exercise does not have to be intense and continuous for physical and emotional benefit. They recommend that "every American adult should accumulate 30 minutes or more of moderate-intensity physical activity over the course of most days of the week" (American College of Sports Medicine, 1993).

Note the word "accumulate." You can effectively improve your health and reduce stress by incorporating activities into your normal daily routine. Examples that can contribute to the 30-minute total are: walking up stairs (instead of taking the elevator), gardening, mowing the lawn, cleaning the house, or planned exercise such as swimming, biking, jogging, or walking. Rather than a regimented exercise routine, you can make many small changes to increase daily physical activity to substantially reduce your risk of developing serious and often costly diseases.

Also note the word "moderate." You need not engage in vigorous, continuous exercise to reap health benefits. Moderate physical activity which we enjoy on a regular basis has a direct impact on both our level of fitness and our level of stress. Russell Pate, President of the American College of Sports Medicine, explained, "The scientific evidence shows that even moderate physical activity can provide substantial health benefits." Dr. Steven Blair, epidemiologist for the Cooper Institute for Aerobics Research, stated that even a little physical activity for the extremely sedentary can reduce the risk of disease as much as smoking cessation (American College of Sports Medicine, 1993).

Rather than intensely push yourself, the latest research says you benefit significantly from such activities as a brisk walk, a swim, a favorite sport, dancing, or raking the leaves. Exercising at a range of 50 percent to 60 percent of the heart's maximum capacity through normal and enjoyable activities that are aerobic, but not very demanding on discipline, results in cardiovascular benefits and reduced stress symptoms. There are more than 26 million adult Americans who enjoy jogging regularly, but if jogging or walking is not for you, there are many other activities to keep you young, healthy, and happy.

If you decide to follow an exercise program rather than accumulate activities towards the daily 30-minute goal, the President's Council (1993d) recommends dynamic movement for 20 minutes or longer, three or more days a week, at an intensity of 60 percent or greater of an individual's maximum heart rate. A workout should include warm-up and cool-down.

Getting Started on Your Exercise Routine

If you are not currently engaged in regular physical activity, begin by incorporating a few minutes of increased activity into your day, building up gradually to 30 minutes a day.

Before you exercise, do a few minutes of warm-ups such as walking in place, arm circles, and knee lifts. Then briefly stretch. After exercising, cool down with a few more gentle stretches. You can use the office stretches presented in Chapter 16 to loosen up or cool down. (I also have a number of other effective, safe stretching routines in my earlier book, *The Fitness Option*.)

Don't be in a hurry to run. It takes patience to get in shape to jog. The Walk Test will help you determine where to begin. If you can comfortably walk three miles in 45 minutes, you are ready to jog, or alternately jog and walk. If you can't pass the test, keep on walking three miles a day until you can do it comfortably in 45 minutes. Set reasonable goals and take care not to overexert.

To enjoy jogging, be sure to take the above steps to avoid injury. You may find it most comfortable to warm up, stretch, and then walk for as long as is comfortable. Using the Walk Test to determine when you are ready to jog, alternately jog and walk for a total of 20 minutes. Walk briskly until you are moving easily. When jogging, speed does not matter. Jog at a comfortable pace until you begin to become winded or tired or both. If you are too breathless to talk, you are going too fast. Walk again until you are ready to jog again. Repeat the cycle until your 20 minutes are up. Once you can run the full 20 minutes, you have completed your conditioning phase, and you can extend your jogging to 30 minutes (President's Council, 1993d).

Cool down thoroughly. Taper off by walking rather than immediately sitting after exercise. Monitor your recovery time. Ten minutes after exercise, you should be breathing comfortably.

Maintain your new fitness level with three workouts a week. Whether you incorporate accumulated moderate physical activity into your day or do a formal exercise routine, you are giving yourself a real fitness and stress reduction treat. Congratulations!

Exercise Prudently

You probably know better than anyone else what your level of fitness is. Are you out of breath from a walk around the block? Are you baffled because the waistbands of your clothes are inexplicably shrinking? Does your lower back ache after any mild activity? These are signals indicating that it's time to make changes. You may have lingering doubts about the safety of exercise, especially if you have never exercised or been physically active before, or have not exercised in a while. Use the following suggestions based on the President's Council and the Cooper Institute's research and experience (Cooper, 1978).

Before starting even a mild exercise program, see your doctor, especially if you are out of shape, have had recent surgery, have high blood pressure, or have any injury such as a torn ligament in your knee which might be stressed by exercise. If you have any history of cardiovascular problems, the President's Council suggests a physician's checkup including an electrocardiogram (ECG). Remember, fitness is an individual quality that varies from person to person, influenced by age, sex, heredity, personal habits, exercise, and eating practices.

───── *BRINGING FITNESS TO THE WORKSITE* ─────

Even with a hectic schedule there are ways to incorporate exercise into your day.

Roy, a computer programmer, is a good example of how it can be done. Roy felt he had too much to do with too little time. He also experienced a buildup of muscular tension in his neck and shoulders due to stress. He felt under constant pressure from his supervisor to "get the job done." Sitting at his computer all day didn't help either. He felt himself "locking up" physically and mentally.

At first Roy resisted the idea of exercise, believing it would take too much time, but we worked out a schedule that fit into his existing commitments. He decided to exercise on the weekend. He liked variety, so on Saturdays he either took his dog for a brisk walk or was physically active with his kids. On Sundays he and his wife walked, biked, or hiked. He also agreed to walk for 20 minutes one day a week at lunch.

For the other four days, he used the "accumulated" moderate physical activity approach. He parked his car in the farthest corner of the parking lot and used the stairs rather than the elevator. Throughout the day he would make a conscious effort to walk. He began using a water cooler at the opposite end of the floor and using a rest room up one flight of stairs rather than the one across the hall. He even ran up and down two flights of stairs on his coffee break. He also did several of the stretching exercises taught in the next chapter.

The results were significant. After a month he reported how much more energy he had, how much clearer his mind was, and how much his muscle tension had been reduced.

With planning you, too, can exercise and get all your work done. Use the following to help pinpoint your options. You may want to combine "accumulated" exercise with a regular exercise routine as Roy did, or use one format or the other alone. Reflect back on your current work stressors. Do you, like Roy, have a sedentary job combined with constant pressure to keep up with a schedule? Has stress on the job resulted in increasing inactivity? Use the space below to describe the situation(s) at work that has led to your lack of exercise and the resulting stress symptoms.

Your work stressor (situational or interpersonal) _____
_____
_____

Your stress symptoms (physical, emotional and/or behavioral) _____
_____
_____

Now make a commitment to regular exercise, whether it be a full workout three times a week or accumulated activities throughout the day. Choose a routine you are willing to try for a month. You can make any needed adjustments after that.

During work hours (for example, a lunchtime jog) _____
_____
_____

Outside work hours (for example, a hike on Sunday) _____
_____
_____

At work accumulated activities (for example, taking the stairs) _____
_____
_____

At home accumulated activities (for example, gardening) _____
_____
_____

There is no substitute for integrating exercise into your daily routine and, for most of us, that means making a conscious effort to bring exercise to the workplace. The next chapter offers effective office stretching exercises for relieving accumulated physical tension while at your desk or workstation.

16

Office Exercises—The Quick Energy Boost

Take a break from your computer. Prevent eye strain, neck and back strain: every 40 minutes stretch, walk around or do relaxation exercises.

—Berkeley Health Letter Associates

Even a few minutes of exercise during the midst of your workday can help enormously in relieving stress. You can easily integrate exercise into your workday effectively and with minimum disturbance. Based on my 25 years of training and teaching experience in ice skating, dance, aerobics, fitness, yoga, and physical therapy, I have developed brief, well-rounded and safe routines well-suited to the relatively sedentary office environment. You can exercise at your worksite even if fitness programs are not offered at your business. Physical exercise is one of the best and quickest ways to release accumulated tensions. Deep, slow breathing, coupled with one or two minutes of stretching exercises, enables contracted muscles to stretch out and relax.

The Sedentary Workplace

Today's high-tech society entices you to be physically inactive. Cars, computers, and labor-saving conveniences have profoundly changed the way people perform their jobs and commute to and from work. Muscle tension can come from simply sitting or standing long hours. Even with an ergonomically correct work station, merely holding one's position for extended periods of time cuts off or slows down circulation in some areas and causes blood to pool in other areas.

On top of a sedentary life style, add deadline pressures, project demands, rush assignments, and budget constraints. This overstimulation expresses itself in our bodies in numerous forms, particularly muscle tension in the neck, shoulders, upper back, and lower back.

Tense (contracted) muscles cause blood to be squeezed out of the tissue, resulting in oxygen and nutrient depletion. Muscle stretching releases tension and increases the flow of oxygen and nutrients into the area. Physical activity and muscle stretching and strengthening release mental and emotional, as well as physical tension.

How to Use the Office Routines

The following routines are designed to activate different muscle groups to give you a complete stretch. They can be practiced sitting at your desk or standing. While these complete routines are recommended, you may feel more comfortable creating your own combinations of stretches. Following each routine, you can select your favorite exercises and put together your own mini-routine to release tension where you feel it most, for example, in your lower back if you sit a lot or your legs if your job involves standing for long periods. However, it is important to stretch your whole body, too, from time to time. After the last routine, suggestions will be provided with the key elements for putting together a full stretch routine that will release tension throughout your body.

When to Stretch

The first routine, for the eyes and hands, is especially beneficial for those who spend a lot of time at a computer or reading. The second set of routines is for tight muscles in the neck, shoulders, and back. The final set focuses on the whole body. Every 30 minutes, do an exercise from routine one and every hour do one of the full routines to prevent a buildup of tension and pain. In between, do one or two stretches any time you feel tension building in any particular area.

To activate different muscle groups, vary which exercises you practice. For example, you might do a few eye exercises, a neck roll, and a side stretch, and an hour later do a shoulder shrug, the hand stimulator, and a sitting cat stretch.

You may need to plan your stretching breaks and provide yourself with a reminder to stop and stretch. For example, you might place a sticky tag on your telephone reminding you to stretch after every call. Or you could place a sticky tag on your computer reminding you to take a Complete Breath and do a shoulder shrug at the beginning of each page or every time you "save" on your computer.

Breathing

As you do the exercises breathe deeply and naturally to a rhythm comfortable for you. For some of the exercises there is a breathing technique at the beginning, as you hold a position, or after the stretch. To briefly review:

1. The Complete Breath—a complete smooth inhalation filling the lungs from bottom to top, and exhaling completely.

2. The Abdominal Breath—inhale, relaxing the abdominal muscles out; exhale, squeezing the abdominal muscles.

3. Three-Part Rhythmic Breath—inhale, hold breath, exhale.

4. Double Breath—inhale through the nose short-long, exhale through the mouth short-long. If you feel you need more practice on the breathing, turn back to Chapter 11.

Good Posture

Throughout the day check your sitting posture. Sitting correctly and comfortably can slow down buildup of tension. To protect your lower back, do not slouch back at the waist. To prevent neck and shoulder strain, do not jut the neck forward. It helps to lengthen the back of the neck by lowering and pushing back your chin. Good posture means to create as much distance as you can from below the navel to the chest. To do this, press your buttocks into the seat of the chair and feel a sense of lengthening the torso up from the anchor of your buttocks and hips.

Contraindications

The exercises release tension from stiff and contracted muscles. Do them at your own pace and to match your needs and limits. If you feel pain in any exercise, stop the exercise. Replace it with another exercise, simplify, or adjust to your physical needs. For example, if you feel any tension arching your neck back, change it by lengthening the back of the neck by pushing your chin back. Do not twist your neck if it is uncomfortable for you. This also applies to your lower back, or any body part that is overly challenged by the exercise. Listen to your body. Make the exercises relaxing and enjoyable.

If you are depressed, it may be difficult to get started. Begin by straightening up your work area, or giving yourself a treat such as some fresh flowers. A cheerful, neat work area helps to lift your spirits. Especially if you are anxious or depressed, bring healthy snacks to work. Avoid sugar and caffeine. The movement and stretching will relax you, improve your circulation, clear your mind, and give you an added boost of energy. It's a wonderful pick-me-up. The results are tangible and immediate! Try it. You will be glad you did.

———— OFFICE ROUTINES #1: FOR EYES AND HANDS ————

Eye Exercises

These eye exercises are especially for those who spend a lot of time reading or at a computer. It strains your eyes to look for long periods at a constant distance and with little eye movement. For good eye health, we need to stretch the eye muscles and look at varied distances. A number of my students at the University of California initially found these exercises hard to do because so much of their time was spent reading. Some found these exercises a good preventative for eye strain-related headaches.

After the exercises give your eyes a short rest—eyes closed, concentrating on relaxing the muscles around the eyes, and allowing the remainder of the body to relax and the mind to quiet. Be attentive to the present moment. When possible, do the eye resting lying down, with a damp, cool cloth over the eyes.

Round-the-Clock

With eyes opened or closed, with a fluid movement look up (twelve o'clock), then circle to the right (three o'clock), then down (six o'clock), and then to the left (nine o'clock). Repeat three more times. Keep the movement flowing and slow—approximately three or four seconds per cycle. Repeat four times counterclockwise. You will feel the muscles stretching. Nice! Rest, with eyes closed, for a Complete Breath.

Big X

With eyes opened or closed, visualize a capital X. Move your eyes from upper left to lower right and back again three times. Follow this by moving eyes from upper right to lower left and back again three times. Take approximately five seconds to do each X—that is, do not rush the movement. Rest, with eyes closed, for a Complete Breath.

Vision Sprinter

Stretch an arm out in front of you at shoulder height, with the hand in a fist and the thumb pointing toward the ceiling. Look at the thumb nail for five seconds (silently count to five); then look across the room, focusing on a more distant point for five seconds; next, look a long distance, if possible, at a point out the window, for five seconds; bring your eyes back to the middle distance for five seconds, and back to the thumb for five seconds. Repeat four times. Rest with eyes closed for a Complete Breath.

Palming

Conclude this series with this soothing exercise. Rub your palms together briskly to generate warmth in your hands, then cover your eyes with your palms. With eyes closed, relax all the muscles around the eyes. Let the warmth penetrate. To deepen the release, visualize the warmth as rays of soothing sunlight streaming into the muscles around the eyes and eyelids.

Hand Stimulator Series

Phase 1: Begin by relaxing your arms by your sides, consciously releasing tension from your shoulders to your fingertips. Now gently twist your hands back and forth from your wrist for five seconds; continue twisting, now from your elbows to your fingertips for five more seconds; continue twisting for five more seconds from your shoulders to your fingertips.

Phase 2: Bring your arms straight out in front of you at shoulder height with your palms facing the floor. Begin by letting your wrists relax down, your hands limp, fingertips toward the floor. Hold for five seconds. Flex back at your wrists, lifting fingertips toward opposite wall, stretching the fingers wide and taut for five seconds. Repeat two more times.

Phase 3: Bend your elbows and bring your hands in front of you at chest height. Without bending at the wrists, spread fingers wide and taut. As rapidly as your can, clench hands into fists and back out, stretching ten times. Relax arms to your sides. Again bend your elbows, hands at chest height, fingers wide and taut. This time just exercise the fingers by squeezing and releasing fingers. Repeat ten times as rapidly as you can.

Finish by repeating Phase 1.

Your Mini-Routines

After practicing Routine #1, you might want to break it up into your own mini-routines scheduled at certain times during your work day. For example:

- 10 a.m.: *Round the Clock; Hand Stimulator, Phase 1; Palming*

- 11 a.m.: *The Vision Sprinter; Hand Stimulator, Phase 2; The Big X.*

Use the space below to put together two mini-routines for the eyes and hands. You might begin with a Complete Breath to relax.

1. _____

2. _____

——— OFFICE ROUTINES #2: FOR NECK, SHOULDERS, AND BACK ———

Below are two routines for the neck, shoulders, and back. One routine is done sitting in a chair. The other is done standing. Read an exercise, practice it once, and then reread the instructions. Once you are familiar with the how-to, each routine takes only a couple of minutes, but be sure to do them in a relaxed manner. It is more beneficial to do a few stretches deeply than to rush through more.

Sitting Vitalizer

Breathing De-Stressor
Sit upright, away from the back of the chair. Take three Double Breaths followed by two Abdominal Breaths.

Sitting Cat
With eyes closed, place your hands on your knees.

A. Tuck your chin and round your spine as much as you can by tightening your abdomen, rounding your back, and curling your shoulders.

B. Now arch your back by rolling your pelvis forward, arching your lower back, and then lifting your chest and chin slightly. Next, reverse to curled position by tucking your chin, curling your chest, and tucking your pelvis again. Repeat the curling and arching three times. Move slowly, consciously, enjoying the stretch.

Sitting Side Stretcher
Continue sitting, with feet hip distance apart, knees bent 90 degrees, chest lifted, abdominal muscles slightly contracted. To help lengthen your spine, feel as if someone is pulling up on the hair on the top of your head. With eyes closed, place your left hand on the edge of your chair. Sweep your right arm in an arc out to the side and then up over your head. Bend slowly to the left. Bend the left elbow only to the degree you want to bend your

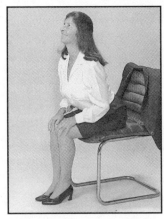
Sitting Cat (A)

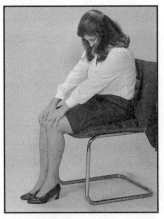
Sitting Cat (B)

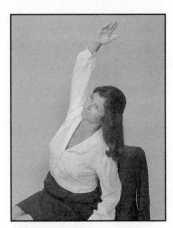
Sitting Side Stretcher

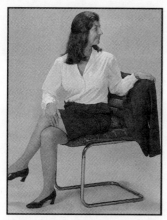
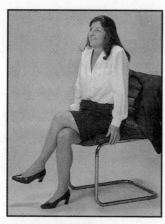

Sitting Spinal Twist   Shoulder Squeeze

trunk to the left. The left hand prevents you from bending too far. Once in the side-stretched position, take two Complete Breaths. As you breathe, think of your right hip and buttocks as an anchor, and feel your right side lengthen and stretch from there. Allow your breath to expand the right ribs by breathing deeply. It feels wonderful. Then bring your trunk upright with your right arm still stretched over your head. Lower your right arm to the side. Repeat to the right side, placing your right hand on the edge of the chair, the left hand overhead then bending to the right.

Sitting Spinal Twist

To release tension in the lower back, sit away from the back of your chair and cross your legs at the thighs. Place your hand along the top outside of the opposite thigh and the other hand on the back of your chair. Look over your back shoulder. Sit with good posture, lifting your chest, lengthening your spine, and pulling your shoulders down. Take three Three-Part Rhythmic Breaths. Turn forward, and repeat to the other side.

Shoulder Squeeze

Lift your shoulders as high as you can, pushing shoulder blades together and squeeze them in toward your ears. Release, relaxing your shoulders down. Repeat two more times.

Standing Tension Eraser

Three-Part Rhythm Breath Movement

Stand with your eyes closed in correct posture. Turn your palms out at your sides, and as you inhale, lift your arms up over your head until your palms touch. Hold your breath, keeping your chest lifted and expanded, your palms pressing together and your shoulders relaxed down away from your ears. As you exhale, lower your hands to your sides. Repeat two more times.

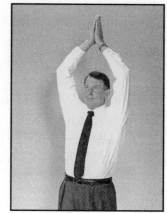

Three-Part Rhythm Breath Movement

Double Breath Movement

Continue standing with your eyes closed and lift your arms up out to the side to shoulder height, with your palms facing forward.

A. Inhale with a Double Breath as you pull your arms back slightly and slightly lift your chin and arch your back.

B. As you exhale with a Double Breath, bring your arms in front of you until the palms touch. At the same time, slightly round your spine, by tucking your chin and bending your knees. From this position, repeat the exercise rhythmically two more times.

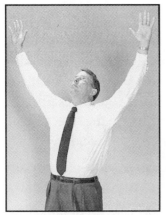
Double Breath Movement (A)

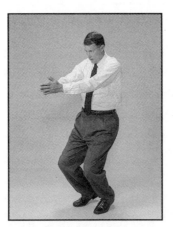
Double Breath Movement (B)

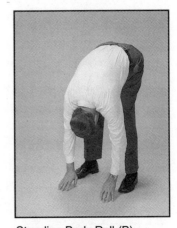
Standing Body Roll (A)

Standing Body Roll

Stand with your feet two feet apart.

A. Lift your chest and chin slightly, gently arch your back, and stretch your arms sideways and upwards at a 45 degree angle.

B. Bend forward, tuck your chin, bring your hands to your shoulders then down your body. Curl your shoulders forward rounding your spine. Partially *bend* your knees, and continue curling all the way down toward the floor. In this rounded, soft position, with your head hanging towards the floor and fingertips resting on or near the floor, take three Complete Breaths. Next, come up slowly, uncurling the spine, stretch your arms sideways and upwards over your head at a 45 degree angle. Gently arch your back, lift chin slightly and press it back, to lengthen rather than arch the back of the neck. Repeat two more times: curling down; holding for

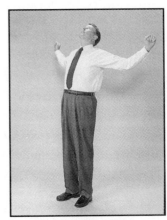
Standing Body Roll (B)

three breaths; and then curling up again. If your hands do not reach the floor, either spread the feet farther apart, or bend over with your hands resting on the seat of your chair. If this is uncomfortable for you, replace this exercise with the Seated Body Roll Exercise in Office Routines #3.

Windmill

Stand with feet hip distance apart, and arms at shoulder height extended out to the sides.

A. As you lower your right arm down and slightly behind you, swing the left arm up and in a clockwise circle across your body at a 45 degree angle to the ceiling. As you twist, let your left heel come off the floor, shifting more of your weight to the right foot. Now reverse the reach and twist, swinging counterclockwise. Repeat to each side two more times.

B. Repeat the Windmill Stretch three more times, this time keeping both arms at shoulder height, again letting the back heel come off the ground.

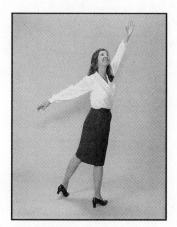
Windmill (A)

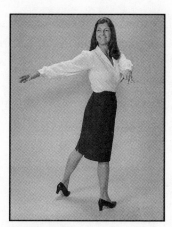
Windmill (B)

Your Mini-Routines

After practicing the Sitting Vitalizer and the Standing Tension Eraser, think about when you might fit them into your day. You could do the sitting routine one day and the standing routine the next. You might prefer to pick out three or four of your favorite stretches from both routines and create your own mini-routine. Or you might add in one of the eye or hand exercises. Choose exercises that release tension wherever you are feeling tight. For example, if you've been sitting all day you might want to stand to release your lower back and increase circulation. The Standing Body Roll and Windmill would be helpful for this.

Choosing your favorite exercises thus far, put together a routine that releases your stress areas.

1. _____

2. _____

3. _____

——— OFFICE ROUTINES #3: FOR THE WHOLE BODY ———

The following two routines, one standing and one sitting, vitalize the whole body. You might want to do them in front of an open window or outside during lunch for an extra boost of energy. Practice each routine, and then, if you prefer, you can create shorter, mini-routines from the exercises described. Each routine takes approximately five minutes to complete. Do remember to relax, breathe deeply, and enjoy.

Standing Full Body Recharger

Arm Circles

Stand with good posture, hands at your sides and take one Complete Breath. Begin by bringing straight arms forward and then over the head. Continue circling, bringing arms back and then downward by the trunk of your body. Repeat two more times. Repeat, circling in the opposite direction.

Continue standing, bringing straight arms, palms up, out to the side, then up over the head until palms touch. Next, lower arms to the side. Repeat two more times. Be sure to breathe deeply and slowly.

Hip Rotations

Stand with feet hip distance apart, with hands on your hips. Rotate your hips in a large circle pivoting the hips like the hands on a clock three times one way and then three times the other way.

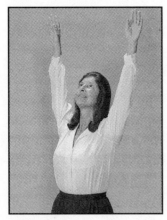
Arm Circles

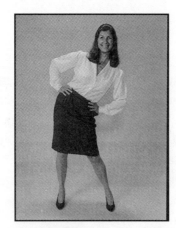
Hip Rotations

Marching in Place

March in place, swinging your arms vigorously, and bending your knees so as to bring them as close to your chest as you can with each step. March lightly for half a minute.

Standing Cat

A. Bend your knees and place your hands on your thighs just above your knees. Round the spine by tucking your chin, and tucking and contracting the buttock muscles.

B. Then arch your spine by pushing your buttocks back, lifting your head, and opening your chest. Repeat, curling and arching with each breath.

Note: If lifting your chin causes tension in the back of your neck, slightly tuck your chin back and down to lengthen back of neck.

Pelvic Tilt

To release tension in your lower back, stand and tilt your pelvis forward by *gently* contracting your buttock muscles and tucking your tail bone. Simultaneously *gently* contract your abdominal muscles in and up toward your chest. Hold for five seconds. Relax muscles for five seconds. Repeat two more times.

To ensure you are doing the Pelvic Tilt correctly, practice once lying on the floor. Lie on the floor with your knees bent. Place your hand behind you on the floor at your waist. Tilt your pelvis as described above. You are doing it correctly if you feel increased pressure against your hand.

The Pelvic Tilt is one of the best exercises you can do to relieve lower back tension. Practice throughout the day, siting or standing.

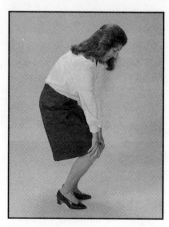

Marching in Place

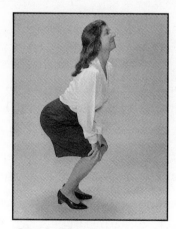

Standing Cat (A)   Standing Cat (B)

Upper Spinal Twist

Keeping your feet hip distance apart and hips not moving, in a pelvic tilt, lift arms in front to shoulder height. Swing both arms as far as you can to the left, with eyes (and head) following the hands. Swing arms to the front again, and repeat to the right side, twisting as far as you can comfortably. Without moving your lower body, swing arms to each side three times. Keep the motion one fluid movement.

Rope Climb

Continue standing. Bring both arms to the side and up over your head, arms parallel, palms facing but not touching. Visualize climbing a rope. As you climb, come up on your toes and stretch up first with one hand and then with the other hand. Feel the stretch from the hips by leaning slightly to each side. Keeping the arms overhead, stretch three times on each side. If you prefer, do not come up on your toes.

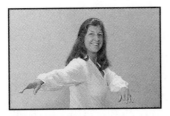

Upper Spinal Twist

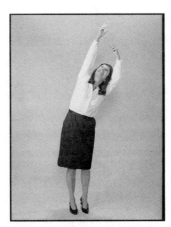

Rope Climb

Relaxer

Sit with spine erect and away from the back of the chair. Take three Complete Breaths, inhaling calmness and peace, letting go more deeply as you exhale completely.

Sitting Full Body Energizer

Seated Body Roll

Sit away from the back of a chair, with your feet parallel, wider than hip distance apart, the back of your heels directly below your knees. Lift your chest and relax your shoulders.

A. To begin, tuck your chin, round your shoulders, curl your spine, and bend forward until your hands reach the floor. Hold this position for one Complete Breath.

B. Come up slowly uncurling the spine and stretch your arms over your head, arching back slightly. Lower your arms. Repeat two more times.

Shoulder Tension Relaxers

A. Sitting upright, curl your shoulders forward, then lift and circle them up toward your ears. Continue to circle, moving your shoulders back and then down. Circle two more times, remembering to breathe deeply. Repeat three more times in the reverse direction—back and up, then forward and down.

B. Alternately lift one shoulder by your ear and then the other. Bring one shoulder up, hold and squeeze the shoulder toward your ear, and then slowly lower the shoulder. Pull the elbow toward the floor for an extra release. Alternately lift, hold, and release each shoulder three times.

Torso Relaxer

Continue sitting, with good posture, feet hip distance apart, knees bent 90 degrees. Bend forward from the hips until you can place your right forearm across your thighs.

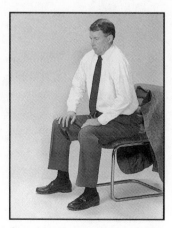

Seated Body Roll (A)

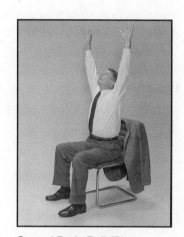

Seated Body Roll (B)

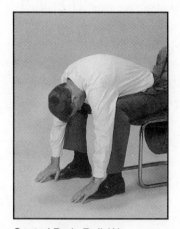

Shoulder Tension Relaxer (A)

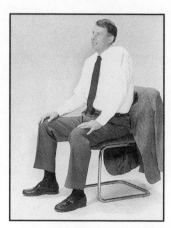

Shoulder Tension Relaxer (B)

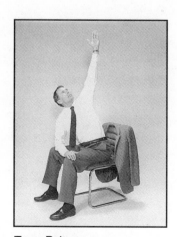

Torso Relaxer

Sweep your left arm over your head, fingers toward the ceiling. Look at the extended hand. Take three Complete Breaths. Let your conscious, deep slow breathing help you be aware of how your body feels. Stay in your comfort zone by listening to your body. If you are not comfortable, skip the exercise or make adjustments. For example, you may prefer to look toward the wall rather than up at your hand. Lower your left arm, and roll back into an upright, seated position. Repeat the stretch and breathing on the other side.

Leg and Buttock Relaxer

Continue sitting away from the back of the chair, feet parallel, hip distance apart, spine upright.

A. Extend and straighten left leg, and flex left heel away from you until leg is parallel to the floor.

B. Point the toes and bend the knee to your chest. Clasp hands around shin and rotate your ankle in a full circular motion, once in each direction.

C. Place left ankle on right thigh just above your knee. To stretch your left buttock, raise your right heel off the floor so that your right knee is higher, and press gently down with both hands on either side of your chair.

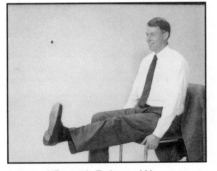

D. For a variation in the stretch, lower right heel to floor, rest your right forearm on your left ankle and your left forearm on your left knee, and bend forward *from the hips* until you feel a stretch in your left buttock. Take three Abdominal Breaths in this position. This stretch is a wonderful lower back relaxer. Repeat to the other side.

Leg and Buttock Relaxer (A)

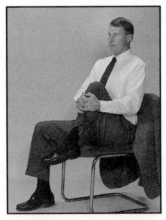

Leg and Buttock Relaxer (B)

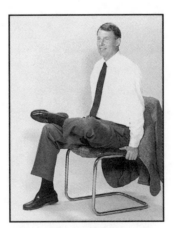

Leg and Buttock Relaxer (C)

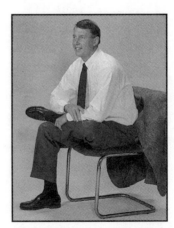

Leg and Buttock Relaxer (D)

Lower Back Releaser

Sit upright in good posture, with legs parallel. Gently twist to the left by taking hold of the back of the chair with your left hand and placing your right hand to the left side of your left knee. Look back over your shoulder. Hold this position for three Complete Breaths. Let each exhalation relax you deeper into the twist. Repeat to the other side.

Nature Breath Relaxer

Take three Three-Part Rhythmic Breaths. With each breath, imagine yourself in your favorite place in nature. Breathe in the fresh air and beauty. Hold the breath and open to your visualization's tranquility and power. As you exhale, mentally and physically release any residual tension.

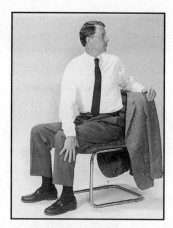
Lower Back Releaser

Your Mini-Routine

If you want to put together your own mini-routine for the whole body, it is important to include those stretches that put your spine through its range of motion. This means:

1. Curling forward and arching back.

2. Stretching to each side.

3. Twisting in each direction—clockwise and counterclockwise.

Choose one exercise from each column to create a routine that puts your spine through its range of motion.

Curling and Arching	Stretching to Each Side	Twisting
Sitting or Standing Cat	Sitting Side Stretcher	Sitting or Standing Spinal Twist
Sitting or Standing Body Roll	Rope Climb	The Windmill
Double Breath Movement	*Torso Relaxer	Lower Back Releaser

*The Torso Relaxer is both a side and twisting stretch.

Valerie's Current Favorite Routine

Here's my own shortened version that includes a stretch from each column and a modification of the Seated Body Roll. I immediately feel the benefits of the exercises I've described. I enjoy them throughout the day, between counseling sessions. I can't imagine not doing them.

Seated Body Roll: (page 112); Rope Climb: (page 112); and the Seated Tension Zapper (below).

Seated Tension Zapper

A. Relax forward with curled spine, as far as is comfortable, hands dangling toward the floor, chest on thighs, neck relaxed. Take two Complete Breaths.

B. Staying bent over, place right hand or fingertips on the floor (or if it feels like too much of a stretch, rest right forearm on your right thigh). Extend your left arm up toward the ceiling and if comfortable look toward the extended left hand. Hold this position for three Complete Breaths. Release arm, and remain curled over. Repeat extension and three breaths on the other side. Come up to a seated position for one Complete Breath.

C. Curl back down, hands relaxed toward the floor. Place your upper arms inside your thighs, elbows near your knees. Place palms together. Now press palms together and simultaneously press your upper arms out against inner thighs and resist with your legs, pushing against your upper arms. Hold for three Abdominal Breaths. Relax for three seconds. Repeat two more times, once with palms facing up, and once with palms facing down. (Varying palm position changes the stretch.)

"Play" with this exercise to adapt it to your body and where you hold your tension. You might curl farther down so that you press farther up on your arms; or lessen your curl so that your lower arms rather than your upper arms press against your thighs.

Now put together your own full-body routine that should take about five minutes to do. Choose three stretches that put your spine through its range of motion, then add others that you enjoy, for example, the Nature Breath Relaxer to release mental tension or Shoulder

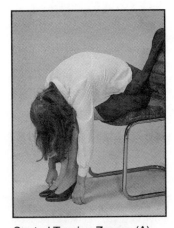
Seated Tension Zapper (A)

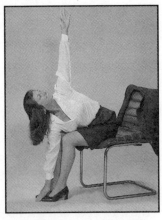
Seated Tension Zapper (B)

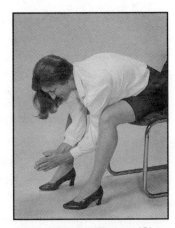
Seated Tension Zapper (C)

Tension Relaxers. The stretches you choose may also depend on the kind of work you do, where in your body you hold tension.

Cheryl, who stands on her feet all day as a clerk in a warehouse, put together the following as her favorite routine. She practiced it two times a day to release her tired legs and lower back and to quiet her mind. First she chose one stretch from each column: Seated Body Roll; Sitting Side Stretch; Sitting Spinal Twist; she then did the Leg and Buttock Relaxer for her lower back; and the arm circles for her neck and shoulders. She ended with three Complete Breaths with her eyes closed.

Angela, who works as a program coordinator for a computer software producer, spends eight hours a day sitting at her desk, on the phone or the computer. Her favorite routine looks very different from Cheryl's. Angela combines mini-routines that rest her eyes, release her neck and shoulder tension, and revitalize her whole body. She also uses a range of spinal motion stretches as the core of her routine. Her routine is:

1. One Complete Breath—seated, eyes closed

2. The Vision Sprinter

3. Palming

4. Shoulder Tension Relaxers

5. Standing Body Roll

6. Rope Climb

7. Windmill

8. Marching in Place

Use the space below to list your own choices appropriate to your work situation and needs.

1. _____

2. _____

3. _____

4. _____

5. _____

6. _____

Throughout the day do one of the mini-routines you created earlier, or even one stretch. Take out five minutes for your newly created favorite full-body routine. Or, you might enjoy doing one of the routines I've put together on the previous pages. All the above are suggestions to maximize benefits, but remember, the best routine is one that you *do*. Relax and have fun—do a spontaneous one any time.

The next chapter deals with another area of wellness that, like exercise, people tend to drop when overstressed at work: healthy eating habits. It will help you get back on track.

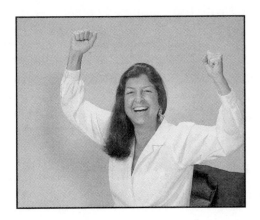

17

Nutrition: Critical Tool for Stress Management

If you can lube your car with it, don't eat it.

—Covert Bailey, *Fit or Fat*

Nutritional common sense during working hours is an excellent tool for building resilience to job stress. With a little creativity and mild self-discipline you can make healthy choices that improve your productivity, your self-esteem, and your waistline.

Nutrition is a vast subject and volumes have been written on it. This chapter focuses on becoming aware of your stress-response eating habits, especially around work, and developing new habits that reduce stress. It presents an optimal nutritional approach for overall stress management including specific tips for healthier eating at work. Gradual, one-step-at-a-time changes result in permanent healthy habits. Apply the turtle and the hare concept and you will come out ahead.

Because of today's emphasis on looking slim, the public is inundated with reducing diets. Rather than concentrating on how to lose weight, let's look at an optimal eating plan for maximizing your vitality and reducing your job stress. This approach to food will also produce a thinner, healthier you.

Note: Integrating dietary changes into your life may or may not be appropriate at this time. Food reflects personal habits and needs. Choose only those suggestions that feel compatible with your approach to nutrition and will aid in reducing your job stress. If a suggestion leads to increased stress, let go of the strategy. One battle plan does not work in all cases. The following recommendations in nutrition have scientific support, but if they do not apply to you, or if they frustrate you, remember, you are the most knowledgeable about what works for you.

Job Stress and Unhealthy Eating Habits

When is the cornucopia of food not overflowing? At all occasions and celebrations the tables are heavily laden with food. Along with the typical three meals a day, there are the frequent gatherings at work: office parties, birthdays, holiday goodies during coffee breaks, and corporate picnics. Not to mention the food served at business lunches and meetings, and coworker wedding and baby showers. Insufficient time is allowed for one meal to digest and assimilate before another morsel is stuffed into the mouth. Given the constant stream of social functions in and outside the workplace, it is a major challenge to maintain a trim waistline and healthful diet.

A common response to the rigors of a full-time work schedule is poor eating habits. Unconscious, out-of-control eating is detrimental to your health, your happiness, and your productivity. This chapter focuses on how to replace work-related unhealthy eating practices. Listed below are typical examples of negative eating habits in response to job stress. Check those that apply to you.

_____ I drink coffee to get going early.

_____ I eat pastries on the run rather than taking the time for a nutritious breakfast.

_____ I drink coffee at work because there is a coffee pot constantly brewing.

_____ I run down to the snack stand in the lobby during a break.

_____ I only have a short time for lunch so I grab a fast food alternative.

_____ I choose fast food because I can't afford a better place to eat.

_____ By afternoon I am exhausted (from all the coffee and being stressed all day). I push myself through the last few hours by snacking on sugary munchies.

_____ I arrive home late after a long commute feeling too exhausted to do the extra work of making a healthy meal. I end up sticking a frozen dinner in the microwave.

_____ After dinner, I watch TV and am tempted by the food commercials. I've had a boring, stressful or difficult day, so I reward myself with a dish of chocolate ice cream.

_____ I go to bed but can't fall asleep due to the chocolate and late-night snacking.

_____ I reward myself with alcohol before, during, or after dinner to release my job stress. As a result, I wake at 3 a.m.

_____ I have a restless night, get up at 5:30 or 6:00 a.m. again and dive for the coffee.

_____ I am groggy at work due to lack of exercise and fresh air.

_____ Other. Add an example of your own.

_____

_____ .

Feeding Your Feelings

Overeating and unhealthy eating reflect the fact that food is more than a means to appease hunger or to enjoy a social or business function. It is deeply rooted in family and social traditions. Since childhood, we have been fed as a reward for doing well, or as an enticement to be good or quiet. For many these beginnings have led to "feeding" a multitude of emotions. When frustrated or angry, disappointed or depressed, excited or bored, one quickly (and often subconsciously) reaches for the cookie jar, a candy bar, or a nibble from the refrigerator. In other words, we feel a positive or negative emotion in response to stress, and feed that emotion with distracted eating. The cause of the emotion does not change, but attention has been momentarily directed away from the problem, and one feels a temporary satisfaction and release through the act of eating.

Four physiological stressors occur when feeding an emotion:

1. Thinking is less clear because blood is directed away from the brain and concentrated in the stomach.

2. The digestive process is less efficient because the parasympathetic nerves which stimulate digestion are slowed by feelings of anxiety and stress.

3. The process of assimilation is overtaxed by the amount of food and its mixed content.

4. There is weight gain due to the type and amount of food eaten. In that emotional moment, usually sugar, chocolate, caffeine, rich pastries, or fast foods are absent-mindedly gobbled.

—— CHARTING YOUR EATING RESPONSES TO JOB STRESS ——

To change these detrimental eating patterns, observe your thoughts. What thoughts and emotions are adversely influencing you to indulge in eating? The following chart will help you see your pattern of eating in response to stress. The next time you find yourself unnecessarily (and often unwillingly) munching, note on the Stress/Food Work Diary what it was that caused you to eat. Some people reach for a cigarette or alcohol; frustrated eating is a similar response to stress.

To attack what I call the stress/food syndrome, first familiarize yourself with how often and regularly you feed an emotion. Are you responding to job stress by nibbling throughout the work day? Or are you barely eating all day and then in the evening stuffing yourself with food as a reward for hard work? Use the daily Stress/Food Work Diary to catch yourself. Keep track until you see your patterns of emotional feeding and its relationship to job stress. Discover which foods you feed to what emotions. This insight allows you to make conscious changes in your behavior.

When I discovered the direct connection between anxiety and cookies, I was shocked by the consistency of the pattern. I reached for the cookie jar every time I felt pressured by a deadline or I didn't know how to fill out a form. It was fascinating to observe myself. It then became amusing. The distancing created by observing but not condemning myself gradually led to a natural change in my behavior. Don't try to force a change. Your observations in themselves will lead to a response which is appropriate for you.

Perhaps you do not respond to stress by feeding your emotions, but instead tend to skip meals. Make sure you note this pattern, too. Erratic eating is hard on your body and your health. Your challenge is to eat regularly despite lack of time or lack of interest.

The following is a sample from a Stress/Food Work Diary to use as a guideline.

Jim, a sports editor for a large city newspaper, used the Stress/Food Work Diary to pinpoint his eating responses to job stress. He knew he'd let his healthy eating patterns slide, but he was surprised when he saw in black and white how off track he had gotten. Below is what he wrote during the first three days of recording in his diary. Use it as an example for filling in your daily diary. Within one week you will clearly see your eating responses to specific job stressors.

Stress/Food Work Diary

	Work Stressor	*Thoughts*	*Emotions*	*Eating Response*
Monday	Rushing to work. Arrive 5 minutes late.	Lousy, rainy weekend! So much work this week! Can't get going.	Fatigue, depression.	2 cups of coffee 2 doughnuts
Tuesday	Busy day. Pizza party at lunch.	I deserve a reward/break.	Uncomfortable socializing at party. Bored, want distraction.	Eat 4 pieces of pizza and Pepsi
Wednesday	Deadline by 4 p.m.	I don't think I can make it. I'll have to push myself.	Anxious, worried.	Skip lunch, drink extra coffee, overeat at night

Stress/Food Work Diary

Monday

Work Stressor	Thoughts	Emotions	Eating Response
_____	_____	_____	_____
_____	_____	_____	_____
_____	_____	_____	_____
_____	_____	_____	_____

Tuesday

Work Stressor	Thoughts	Emotions	Eating Response
_____	_____	_____	_____
_____	_____	_____	_____
_____	_____	_____	_____
_____	_____	_____	_____

Wednesday

Work Stressor	Thoughts	Emotions	Eating Response
_____	_____	_____	_____
_____	_____	_____	_____
_____	_____	_____	_____
_____	_____	_____	_____

Thursday

Work Stressor	Thoughts	Emotions	Eating Response
_____	_____	_____	_____
_____	_____	_____	_____
_____	_____	_____	_____
_____	_____	_____	_____

Friday

Work Stressor	Thoughts	Emotions	Eating Response
_____	_____	_____	_____
_____	_____	_____	_____
_____	_____	_____	_____

Changing Your Eating Responses to Job Stress

Now that you see your stress/food syndrome patterns, you can make changes that are easy to do, quick, and healthy. The following list will give you ideas.

1. Supply your kitchen and office with healthy, easily available snacks.

2. Thirst is often masked as hunger—keep juices and teas handy.

3. Regularly drink water to reduce snacking. Keep a water bottle at your work station.

4. Eat a nutritious breakfast—blend your own energy-booster drink of juice, banana, nonfat yogurt, and protein powder, or create a combination of your choosing. Or have an easy-to-fix whole wheat toast or bagel with peanut butter and fruit-sweetened jam. Or have an apple or banana with a muffin. You have time for these quick fixes.

5. Bring your lunch to work. Make a sandwich of whole grain bread, low-fat mayonnaise and low-fat fillings such as tuna packed in spring water. Be creative—use cilantro and dijon mustard to flavor, and add mushrooms, red bell peppers, and sprouts.

6. Bring nutritious foods to microwave for lunch. Use leftover rice or pasta with pre-steamed vegetables. Use low-sodium soy sauce or tamari to flavor.

7. Make dinners with one portion extra to microwave at lunch the next day.

8. For a sweet tooth keep naturally sweetened cookies available.

9. For bulk—keep flavored nonfat rice cakes handy. These fill you up without the calories or fat. Try air-popped popcorn with curry or soy sauce.

Alternative Mood Foods

Your moods influence your choice of foods. It is conversely true that you can influence your moods by what you eat. Specific foods can stimulate or calm.

Foods containing an amino acid called tryptophan stimulate serotonin, which calms and increases concentration. Foods containing the amino acid tyramine stimulate production of norepinephrine and dopamine, which give you a boost when fatigued. Eat a small amount of protein to increase energy and alertness and a small amount of carbohydrates as a natural tranquilizer.

10. Power Lunches and Snacks. Choose low-fat, protein-rich foods to increase motivation, reaction time, and alertness. When you have plans for a busy afternoon, or need an extra boost to finish the day's projects, eat a lunch high in protein or

have a late afternoon snack of no more than three to four ounces of lean beef, skinned chicken, fish, or a low-fat dairy product, or a "power" candy bar.

11. After Work. Before bedtime, have a carbohydrate such as an oatmeal cookie or bite of pasta to induce a sleepy, relaxed mood. Warm food, such as tea with honey, or a warm muffin, not only provides the carbohydrate, but also gives a sense of nurturing and security. Have no more than one to two ounces of the carbohydrate for the desired effect, and to prevent weight gain, make low-fat selections. For those who are 20 percent or more over their ideal weight or for women a few days prior to menstruation, two to three ounces may be required.

Use the Stress/Food Work Diary to become aware of the types of food you crave when stressed. Types of food are often related to the type of mood you are experiencing. When feeling bored or in need of nurturing, do you consume soft, creamy foods such as custards and pastries? When you are angry or frustrated, do you reach for chewy, hard foods such as nuts or popcorn?

12. Replace mood foods with nutritious, nonfat selections that are similar in texture to the foods that match your emotion.

13. Keep crunchy celery, carrots, and apples on hand for biting into resentment or anxiety.

14. Turn to nonfat, plain yogurt with honey or a cup of hot tea for lonely times.

15. Use the office microwave for cooking a low-fat warm entree to soothe yourself emotionally at lunchtime.

Alternative Activities

Once you have adjusted what you eat, you can elect to go one step further: changing your response to stress. Rather than eating, engage in an activity that releases your tension.

At first you may find yourself doing the stress-reducing technique and eating too. Observe the process, and then, just once, use discipline to stop yourself from eating. Use this one time as a starting point from which to drop the stress/food syndrome.

Before your next bout with the stress/food syndrome, practice several stress-releasing options that would be appropriate to your situation and time available.

1. Take three Three-Part Rhythmic Breaths.

2. Go for a one-minute to twenty-minute walk.

3. Do some slow, deep stretches.

4. Close your eyes and affirm, "Peace *(strength, courage, love)* within brings peace *(strength, courage, love)* without."

5. Jog in place.

6. Tense and relax all your muscles three times.

7. If the emotion is a low-energy emotion like depression, release the stress with an activity that gently raises your level of energy (for example, one of the office exercises from Chapter 16), or walk down the hall or to the restroom.

8. It's helpful to get outside and breathe fresh air.

9. Find a spot outside to stretch, breathe, and relax.

10. If your stress is expressed as a high-energy emotion such as anger, do an initial active release such as running up the office stairs or briskly walking around the parking lot.

11. Follow this with one of the calming techniques. Create your own new responses and practice them.

12. Visualization can be very helpful in this situation. At your work station, take one minute to sit with eyes closed. Take several breaths and then visualize a situation to which you previously responded by eating. Now replace that image. See yourself expressing a new, non-eating response to stress. Practice this visualization several times a day and allow yourself to carry it out.

You can beat the typical "indulgence" food response to job stress using the two above lists of alternative eating habits and alternative activities. In the exercise below choose possible alternatives you are willing to practice from the lists above and add your own creative ideas. Dorothy, a claims adjuster for an insurance company, used this exercise to come up with healthier ways of coping with her job stress. Use her first three listings to help get you started.

You are changing direction, turning yourself around from a life of anxiety to one of well-being. Initially this takes extra effort and preparation. Once you stop the downhill slide, the walk up the hill is expansive and more exhilarating with each step. You may backslide and find your hand in the cookie jar, but if you see the climb up as two steps forward, one step back, or as a zigzag, you will realize that the direction and momentum are still up. One backslide is not a change in direction, it just sets the pace of the upward climb.

I have discussed changing what you eat and/or substituting a stress-releasing skill as a response to your stressors. Perhaps you have tried this before, or it is not helpful for you. If so, try another approach. Rather than working on changing your response to your emotions, go back to the Stress/Food Work Diary and note the emotions you are experiencing. Look for negative thoughts you hold that are causing the emotions. Perhaps you can change your attitude to a situation or towards a person. Or is there anything you can do to change the situation itself? Chapters 18 and 19 give you methods for changing negative thinking patterns and improving communications. If you still cannot get to the root of the

Nutrition

Stress/Emotions	Alternative Foods	Alternative Activities
Bored	Fruit juice/fruit	Stretching exercises
Lonely	Yogurt, tea	Talk to a coworker or get outside
Angry	Apples, carrots	Run up the stairs; go on an errand
_____	_____	_____
_____	_____	_____
_____	_____	_____
_____	_____	_____
_____	_____	_____
_____	_____	_____
_____	_____	_____
_____	_____	_____
_____	_____	_____
_____	_____	_____
_____	_____	_____
_____	_____	_____
_____	_____	_____
_____	_____	_____
_____	_____	_____
_____	_____	_____

problem, perhaps the ideas below on compulsive eating will give you some ideas for positive change.

Compulsive Eating and Low Self-Esteem

If you handle stress by compulsive eating, it may mean you are running away from facing your emotions by stuffing or suppressing them. Feeding a deep sense of lack produces a vicious cycle of overeating followed by sugar and fat cravings, which never result in fulfillment. Perhaps you race through life actively reaching outside yourself for happiness to avoid looking at a past trauma or a current pain. Keeping constantly busy, filling spare moments with eating, masks inner suffering.

Normally, eating as a response to stress results in overweight. The increasing bulge becomes an embarrassing sign of emotional turmoil. Weight due to compulsive eating becomes especially harmful when overeaters internalize the embarrassment of a pudgy body into a shame of their very existence. Whether or not low self-esteem initiated the eating response to stress, the resulting overweight usually leads to acute devaluation of the self.

Recently, I had the heartbreaking experience of witnessing this process. An obese client and I decided to sit in a sunny meadow for our counseling session. As we sat down, I adjusted my chair two inches away from her because the uneven ground caused my chair to wobble. Her immediate reaction was to assume I moved back because I could not bear to be near her. Anger at herself for not being able to break her habit of overeating had become distorted into feelings of low self-worth and depression.

Authors John Bradshaw and Joan Borysenko state that there are two types of shame. Healthy shame results in taking responsibility for the outcome of a behavior and changing that behavior, or accepting the consequences of that behavior (overweight). Unhealthy shame results from turning an external act into an internal debasing of the self. This process often begins in childhood. Devalued in childhood by conditional love and psychological abuse or neglect, the adult now carries a "wounded child within" who needs emotional nurturing, not external feeding. Most of us carry a "wounded child within." Our self-esteem and view of the world around us as friendly or unfriendly is largely a reflection of the degree of nurturing and unconditional love we received as children (Bradshaw, 1990; Borysenko, 1987).

Look at your past and search out possible unfulfilled needs of childhood. Perhaps compulsive eating is a response to childhood abandonment, a feeding of childhood loss and loneliness. Changing eating patterns will not solve the problem because the roots are deep. Past abuse, neglect, family alcoholism, and skewed family situations result in misconceptions about oneself and the universe. Often, past rejection by significant others has been internalized as lack of self-esteem and alienation from the surrounding world. This negative self-image may be expressed in dysfunctional eating patterns.

If this describes your situation, counseling or a support group may be needed to help you break the cycle of low self-esteem and compulsive eating. Apply the suggestions in this book, but if you need more support, seek out professional help (see Chapter 24).

One last suggestion for self-help is to take responsibility for fulfilling unmet childhood needs yourself. Rather than reaching out, expecting others to meet your needs, meet them yourself. You understand where you feel an inner lack and what is needed to fill the void. Nurture yourself with something other than food, like a bubble bath or massage. Your "wounded child within" needs your love and parenting. The essence of who you are has been injured and needs your unconditional caring and support. You might reward yourself each week with a little something special just for you, perhaps a bouquet of flowers or a plant for your desk.

One client, after many years of unsuccessful relationships, saw that she counted on her job to make her happy. Rather than taking responsibility for her own happiness, she relied on her coworkers to fill the lonely void within. This pressure on her coworkers caused constant friction. With counseling, she began to accept herself, and to accept time at home alone as a private healing time, rather than as a time of remorse and proof that she was unworthy of love. As she gained her own independence and self-appreciation, she became a less needy and demanding coworker.

Creating Your Stress Management Diet

Moderation is the building block of sound nutrition and a stress-free diet. What you eat day-to-day is important, not the Friday night heavy meal or the once-a-week rich dessert. Restricted diets take the pleasure and relaxation out of eating. Eat with awareness, watch calories, salt, fat, and cholesterol intake without the stress of complete denial.

Stress-free eating means observing daily patterns and making minimal but consistent changes towards healthy nutrition. As you did at the beginning of this chapter, the first step is to become aware of your eating habits without changing them, and observe the physical, mental, and emotional effects of your current diet. The most effective way to change the unhealthy aspects of your diet is to see change as directional and to view it within the framework of long rhythms. To avoid stress, remember that the *process* of working toward an ideal is more important than the goal itself. Do not set restrictions to be endured for a specific amount of time; instead make incremental changes within the framework of a lifetime direction of healthy eating.

There is no diet that is right for everyone. It only creates stress to follow someone else's ideal diet. Dieting in itself is stressful because of the built-in nature of an outside authority dictating what you eat. Balance enjoyment with healthful eating and observe nutritional habits that work for you. Changes do not happen overnight. Learn to listen to your body to discover its nutritional requirements. Consult a nutritional practitioner if you are not sure how to correct an imbalance in your system.

Nutritional Tips for Reducing Stress

In creating your stress management diet, making even small changes using one or more of the following suggestions will enhance your vitality and reduce your stress symptoms. For those who relieve stress through overeating, the changes will also help you to reduce weight.

1. Eat more fruits and vegetables. A salad once a day is excellent for your health. Raw salads are not only rich in vital nutrients, but give you fiber to help in elimination. Green leafy vegetables are an excellent source of calcium, which the body demands when under stress.

2. Eat as much fresh food as you can. The more processed the food, the less vitality available to you. A bowl of fresh fruit is much better for you than a bowl of canned fruit. If your tension expresses itself as indigestion, light meals with emphasis on fruit alone or vegetables (do not eat them at the same meal) can work wonders. If you have trouble digesting raw foods, lightly steam or bake them. Add a little water to sliced fruit such as apples, bananas, and pears and simmer for a warm, easy-to-digest breakfast on a cold, winter day.

3. Begin to shift from demineralized cereals, white flour, and white rice to whole grain breads and grains. Stress robs your body of nutrients, especially the B vitamins, which are called the anti-stress vitamins. Whole grains and breads are rich in these important vitamins. Nutritional yeast is an excellent source of B vitamins and can be sprinkled in soups (homemade, if possible) or on salads, or added to casseroles. If you are allergic to wheat, try some of the delicious sprouted breads which have no wheat in them, or bread made with corn.

4. When you're under stress, your immune system is weakened. Vitamin C is essential for proper functioning of the adrenal and thyroid glands and "promotes healing in every condition of ill health" (Airola, 1981). Good sources of vitamin C are citrus fruits and juices and all fresh fruits and vegetables, especially broccoli, tomatoes, bell peppers, apples, and kiwis. Eat some of these daily or have a large raw salad.

5. Avoid sugar, by the teaspoon or hidden in processed foods. For example, there are eight tablespoons of sugar in a twelve-ounce serving of Pepsi or Coca-Cola. In terms of stress management, sugar gives you an initial burst of energy, but is followed by a low-energy, depressed feeling, because it upsets the balance in your blood sugar level.

6. Avoid or cut down on caffeine in coffee, black teas, soft drinks, and chocolate. Caffeine draws the B vitamins out of the body. After the initial stimulus, you have less energy. Ask those who have given up coffee and they will tell you they have more energy and less of the pendulum swing of energy to lethargy. See Appendix

A, Caffeine Chart, for list of substances high in caffeine. Reduce the amount of coffee you drink, or mix it half and half with decaffeinated coffee; or, if possible, give it up entirely. You will be surprised how much better you feel. I drank one cup of coffee a day for a year. At about 4 p.m. every day I was exhausted. I now maintain as full a schedule as before and I am tired at the end of the day, but it is a natural tiredness not the exhaustion I felt before quitting my one cup of coffee.

7. Eat three meals a day. This is essential. Stress is exacerbated by irregular eating patterns.

8. Make rich meals and desserts a treat rather than a daily habit. Have a small piece of lasagna or chocolate mousse, but then keep the next meal light, with an emphasis on fiber.

9. A general rule is to eat those foods that give you energy yet do not tax the system. The answer lies in eating fresh, live foods in correct combination so as to aid digestion, assimilation, and elimination.

Nutrition is as controversial as politics and religion, with countless books and theories on what is healthy. For stress management, the above tips are guidelines. The essential rules are moderation, common sense, and a diet that is both enjoyable and healthy for you.

A Healthful, Highly Disciplined, Low-Fat Diet

If you want to delve into another approach, the following is a healthful, highly disciplined diet which has had success in battling illness, in aiding in stress reduction, and in reducing weight. Consult your physician before making any significant changes in your nutritional patterns. This more stringent regimen has been very beneficial for some people, but it may not be best for you. It is a low-fat (optimally less than 20 percent) vegetarian diet with emphasis on fresh (organic, if possible) foods. This diet has no fish, chicken, or red meat, no eggs, and only low-fat dairy products. It includes only those foods listed below.

- Fresh fruits and vegetables
- Whole grains: *especially brown rice, oats, millet, and buckwheat*
- Legumes: *best sprouted to increase vitamin and mineral content*
- Dairy products: *focus on low-fat milk and yogurt, and soft cheeses or the new low-fat hard cheeses*
- Herbal teas *such as peppermint, chamomile, and lemon verbena*
- Honey or fruit juices *for sweetening, rather than sugar*
- Fresh fruit and vegetable juices

To maintain such a diet, eat hearty meals that emphasize the food itself rather than the condiments under which the food is usually buried. For example, to keep to the low-fat aspect of the diet, use one of the no-oil salad dressings on the market or create your own. I use a little vinegar and vegetable broth with brewer's yeast. Or you could use a squeeze of lemon, mashed avocado, and herbs. Skip the butter on vegetables, including corn and potatoes, or use a little of the monosaturated oils such as olive oil.

To keep the fat down, do not use mayonnaise in sandwiches; instead, try the following nonfat yogurt spread. Take several tablespoons of nonfat plain yogurt and place it in the refrigerator overnight in a strainer covered with cheesecloth, or in a coffee filter paper or a paper towel. The next morning toss away the drained liquid collected in the pan below the strainer and flavor the resulting yogurt spread with your favorite spices. I use this on potatoes and sometimes in salads.

Use egg substitute or egg whites in your baking. If you are new to vegetarianism, ask your local health food store for a good cookbook. Foreign cuisines, such as Chinese, Mexican, and Italian, have many non-meat entrees which are easy to prepare. I have been a vegetarian for over 25 years and highly recommend that you give it a try for stress reduction and healthy living.

This low-fat vegetarian diet can be tailored to fit what you and your physician feel is best for you. The American Cancer Society and the American Heart Association recommend a low-fat diet (maximum 30% fat) and cutting back on red meat because of its high

How much fat is in the foods you eat?

IT ISN'T HARD TO FIGURE OUT how much fat is in the foods we eat. But it's almost impossible just by looking at the label! Often, fat content is listed in grams or milligrams. But what you need to know is "What percentage of the calories in this food come from fat?" The simple mathematical formula in this chart will help you to watch out for your fat consumption.

Step One

Grams of Fat (Per serving)	x	9 (Calories/gram)	=	Calories from Fat

Step Two

Calories from Fat (per serving)	÷	Total Calories (Per serving)	=	Percentage of Fat (in food)

FOR EXAMPLE: In whole milk, the label lists 8 gm of fat per serving. Multiply that by 9 and you get 72 calories from fat per serving. Divide that by 150 (the total calories per serving) and you get 48%. **In short, 48% of the calories in whole milk come from fat!**

cholesterol. These sources say you should eat a maximum 300 milligrams of cholesterol per day. If you do not know the percentage of fat in a food you are eating, the previous chart will help you. Find the percentage of fat in a product by multiplying the number of grams of fat by nine and then dividing the result by the total calories. The number of calories and amount of fat are listed on packaged food.

The current labeling on packaged foods can be confusing. The labeling states the total calories and fat calories, but only gives the percentage of fat calories based on Daily Values (DV) of 2,000 calories. This is based on total consumption of fat for the day, not the individual serving percentage of fat. (This is helpful if you total your calories each day, but confusing if you want to know the percentage of fat per serving.) For example, the label for one cup of whole milk states: "Total fat 8 grams, DV 12% Fat." Using the previous chart, you learn a cup of milk is 48% fat!

A general rule of thumb for controlling cholesterol intake is to avoid saturated fats and reduce consumption of animal products such as red meat and dairy products, including butter and eggs.

Using Nutritional Guidelines at Work

Let me again emphasize that nutrition can play a significant role in reducing stress only if it is carried out with knowledge and enthusiasm. Take your first steps with a suggestion or two from this chapter, and gradually make changes only when you feel ready to enjoy the results.

To summarize, essential nutritional tools of stress management are

1. Eat sensibly, particularly eat fresh fruits and vegetables, whole grains and legumes, and foods low in fat, cholesterol, and sugar.

2. Eat three regular meals a day and try not to eat after dinner.

3. During working hours act consciously when you eat; don't snack absentmindedly, drink caffeine all day, or skip meals. This will stabilize your blood sugar, reduce your weight, and help you cope with stress.

4. If you are feeding your emotions rather than your hunger, gradually change what you eat from processed, fat- and sugar-laden foods to satisfying, healthy foods.

5. Attempt to change your response to stress from one of eating to an alternative stress-reducing activity.

6. Above all, the process of changing nutritional habits needs to be in gradual steps, with an eye to moderation.

You can greatly reduce job stress both by changing your attitudes and thoughts and by changing your situation with improved communication skills. The next two chapters on these topics give you the means to reduce the negative emotions you have been feeding.

18

Reframing Your Thinking Patterns

*The secret of overcoming feelings of guilt is to view your mistakes
as prods, merely, to ultimate victory.*

> —J. Donald Walters, *The Secret of Overcoming
> Harmful Emotions*

*The secret of happiness lies not in events but in our response
to them.*

> —Barry Neil Kaufman,
> *Happiness is a Choice*

As a friend of mine says, "Stress begins between the ears." How we think directly affects our moods. Negative thinking produces negative moods; positive thinking produces positive moods. It's that simple! Thus, the essence of stress is not found in the circumstances surrounding us; rather, it is found in our *response* to them. As Shakespeare said, "There is nothing either good or bad, but thinking makes it so" (*Hamlet* Act II, Scene ii.) And, as the Chinese proverb says, "Change your thoughts, and you change the world." Life may be painful or unfair, but it is a cognitive choice to paint it a disaster or catastrophe. We can learn how to paint life in positive and manageable terms.

Your *perceptions*—not any objective reality—govern your emotional response and resulting behavior. Perceptions are based on beliefs, assumptions, values, and conditioning. You can dramatically reduce stress by changing your distorted perceptions. You can remove anger, anxiety, or depression by changing the thoughts that create the emotion.

For example, Barbara's distorted thinking exaggerated her shortcomings and led to agitation and defeatism regarding her ability to successfully complete a project. Changing her self-talk from "This is way over my head" to "I'll give it my best shot" changed her gloom into excited anticipation and enthusiasm. Like Barbara, we often paint events much worse than they actually are by our distorted thinking. This greatly increases our stress.

The previous chapters focused on ways to relax your body and quiet your mind. In the last chapter you learned how stress can trigger unhealthy eating habits. This chapter concentrates on ways you can consciously alter your negative thinking patterns. Changing distorted perceptions that fuel negative emotions is an essential and effective stress management tool.

A Hardiness Personality Reduces the Impact of Stress

What is the impact of changing one's perspective of a situation? Research on stress has found that "psychological hardiness" decreases the chances of becoming ill due to stress by as much as 50 percent (Witmer and Sweeney, 1992). According to these studies, *developing optimism* (seeing life's stressors as challenges rather than obstacles), *increasing commitment* (becoming involved in life rather than feeling separate and alone), and gaining a sense of *control, empowerment, or competence* (versus feeling the victim in highly stressful situations) make the difference between coping with life or being overwhelmed by it. Developing a "Hardiness Personality" with these qualities decreases the probability of illness (Witmer and Sweeney, 1992).

You can change a negative attitude toward yourself or toward the world into a positive, life-affirming attitude. To change your thinking habits, you need to challenge old, habitual patterns of thought. But before you can change limiting or detrimental thoughts, you need to become aware of your thought patterns. The following techniques are proven, constructive methods for becoming aware of your thought patterns and empowering yourself in relation to your thoughts. The four-step exercise is designed to help you free yourself of distorted thinking and its stressful impact.

HOW TO CHANGE NEGATIVE THINKING IN FOUR STEPS

Step 1. Become aware of negative self-talk.

Carry a pen and a small notebook with you to work. As often as feasible, even if only once a day, write down your negative thoughts for at least a week. Writing at the same time each day, such as on your afternoon break, helps make this exercise a habit. Are your statements pessimistic? Are you viewing yourself as ineffectual, seeing a situation as an obstacle rather than a challenge? Do your statements imply you are withdrawing rather than becoming involved in life? For one week write down your negative thoughts, attitudes, and resulting emotions in the following four column format.

In the first column write negative statements about yourself. These thoughts could be self-blame, guilt, or other negative judgments. In the second column write negative statements about the world around you. In the third column note what attitudes or perceptions your statements in columns one and two express. In the fourth column label the negative emotion you are experiencing due to your perception of the situation. This exercise dramatically reveals the relationship between your negative thoughts and your negative emotions. How are your attitudes different from the Hardiness Personality attitudes of commitment, self-empowerment, and optimism? The following is an example of how to use the chart on the following page.

Henry, a budding architect in a small New York firm, was praised by his boss for a just-completed project. He had expected a raise, but when the raise did not materialize, Henry felt hurt. The following shows how his negative inner talk resulted in bitterness and disappointment.

Rather than accepting the praise at face value and taking it as encouragement, Henry allowed his negative self-talk to cloud an otherwise positive situation.

Henry's Self-Talk Awareness Diary

My Negative Self-Talk About Myself	My Negative Self-Talk About the World	My Perception	My Emotions
I never seem to do anything well enough.	The boss is only saying he likes my work or he would have given me a raise.	I don't belong here.	Bitterness Hurt Disappointment

Self-Talk Awareness Diary			
My Negative Self-Talk About Myself	*My Negative Self-Talk About the World*	*My Perception*	*My Emotions*

Step 2. Replace distorted thoughts.

Your thoughts are influenced by your past. Childhood experiences color your present level of self-esteem. A nurturing childhood, with age-appropriate expectations, builds a higher level of self-confidence than one filled with unrelenting criticism, lack of caring, or unrealistically high expectations. Constant faultfinding, or pressures created by rigid, perfectionist demands from a parent, sibling, or teacher cast a shadow of self-doubt which darkens adult self-worth. A difficult challenge becomes a bewildering obstacle if you have low self-esteem. You become your harshest critic by internalizing the negative judgments of others.

Rather than blame a person or situation for your low self-worth, improve your self-esteem by curtailing limiting thought patterns. These include judgmental statements regarding yourself or others.

Common Thinking Distortions

The following list consists of common thought distortions (Burns, 1980). Look at your diary of self-talk for the week at work. Do you recognize any of these distortions in your thoughts and perceptions?

☐ 1. **Black and White Thinking.** When you make a mistake, do you declare yourself a failure? If so, you have perfectionist, unrealistic expectations that result in guilt, frustration, and depression. Remember, you are a success every time you learn from a mistake!

☐ 2. **Tunnel Vision.** Do you only see the negative aspect of a situation, person, or yourself? Do you discount positive aspects of yourself, an event, or others to uphold your negative, distorted view? Do you tend to select information which substantiates your perception, ignoring contrary facts? Judgment muddies the broader picture.

☐ 3. **Negative Interpretation**. Do you, without questioning or clarifying, assume someone else has a negative attitude toward you? If so, you predict a negative outcome of a situation and act on that "reality."

☐ 4. **Exaggeration**. Do you minimize your assets and others' faults, and magnify your faults and others' assets? A difficult circumstance becomes a catastrophe.

☐ 5. **Personalization**. Do you blame yourself for a situation that is not primarily your fault? You inappropriately take responsibility for events beyond your control.

Learn these five categories of distortions so you can catch yourself in the act of distorting! Never mind *why* you do it, just change the thought to a more rational, neutral, or expanded view. Recognizing the fallacy of your distortions robs them of their power. This will improve your self-esteem and reduce your stress.

Now use the following four-column technique to attempt to replace your distorted self-talk with a more neutral or positive view. Drawing upon your diary or a current work stressor, describe the situation that caused you to be stressed in the first column.

In the second column write your negative self-talk about yourself. In the third column write your negative self-talk regarding the situation or other people involved in the event. Use the fourth column for writing a replacement for each distorted or negative thought. Think of what a friend, counselor, or person you respect might say. Is there a counterpoint to your negative perspective? A glass that is half empty may also be viewed as half full, or as both half full and half empty. Talk back to your negative statements. If you do not replace/answer a negative statement, one negative thought leads to the next, in a downward spiral.

Do this powerful exercise for a week. Below is an example to guide you.

George was astounded. Sarah, his accountant for many years, had made the nightly bank deposit for his flourishing toy store without enclosing the deposit slip. A loss of $1,597.00!

George's Positive Thought Replacement Chart			
Trigger Situation	*Negative Self-Talk About Myself*	*Negative Self-Talk About Situation/Others*	*Positive Thought Replacement*
Deposit without deposit slip.	I was a fool to trust her. I'm a poor judge of character.	She is totally irresponsible. The bank must think we are incompetent.	Well, no money was lost. She has always been responsible. This is her first big error. She has appeared distracted lately. Perhaps I need to talk to her.

Before doing your own Positive Thought Replacement Chart, identify the thinking distortions in the above example. Then review your own Self-Talk Awareness Diary for distortions.

1. Using the list of Common Thinking Distortions, write a "G" beside each of those you see George using in the example above. "She is totally irresponsible" is, for example, Exaggeration.

2. Go back over your own Self-Talk Awareness Diary. Place your initial by your thinking distortions.

Positive Thought Replacement Chart			
Trigger Situation	*My Negative Self-Talk About Myself*	*Negative Self-Talk About Situation/ Others*	*Positive Thought Replacement*

3. Using the lists of Common Thinking Distortions, place a check mark by those you have observed yourself using.

Recognizing clearly the ways you are inaccurately viewing a situation will help you to create a more accurate statement to replace it.

Step 3. If you can't change it, accept it; if you can change it, do so!

Now look again at your trigger situations. If a situation cannot be changed, either accept it or change your view of it. This perceptual shift will lift your spirits, and free you from the prison of emotional stress. It helps to list the positives of seemingly black circumstances. Focus on what *does* work, rather than on the negatives.

If you find fault in a situation, is there anything you can do about it? Rather than criticize, begin to think in terms of taking action. If feasible, begin to turn your negative energy towards positive solutions. Your involvement may make a difference even indirectly to improve a situation and reduce your own stress in the process. Many inspiring stories originate from people who cared enough to make an effort to change a situation. I remember an article about a postman who saved all year to buy mittens for the homeless. Each Christmas season his caring gesture of offering gloves to any passer-by made for warm hearts as well as warm hands. His Hardiness Personality qualities of involvement and commitment strengthened his ability to cope with his own stressful issues.

> *Michael is a client who came to me complaining of depression. He had grown despondent largely because his office had no windows, he worked alone and felt isolated. First we worked out some tangible changes: setting up full spectrum lighting in his office, initiating walks at lunch with coworkers, and commuting by bicycle. Then he worked on recognizing the advantages of his room. He started to see it as a quiet, private place where he could work at his own pace. He became enthusiastic again by both taking responsibility for making changes and reframing his perception of his situation.*

Like Michael, can you change your view of a negative work situation? Is there anything you can do or say to make it tolerable? Observe how you feel emotionally and physically when you have more positive thoughts. By changing your attitude, for example, from "I can't stand it" to "Well, I may not like it, but . . . " reduces agitation and/or a sense of being overwhelmed. The situation does not change but your acceptance of what you cannot change reduces your stress. You can get a better night's rest!

Step 4. Create a positive environment for yourself.

It helps tremendously to have reinforcement as you work on your thinking patterns. Our thoughts are deeply affected by the people we spend time with and how we make use of our leisure time. Coworkers, a counselor, or a support group can help you through the rough times. Decide to take a walk at lunch with someone who is positive about the job or enthusiastic about their own lives. They will have a favorable impact on your thinking. See Chapter 20 on Social Support for further suggestions.

Notice who and what situations drag you back into old negative thought patterns. Use discrimination regarding what you talk about during a coffee break. You can redirect a nonproductive, negative conversation.

Books, television, and movies also greatly impact our thoughts and resulting moods. Be selective. To increase awareness of the powerful effect of environment, use your notebook to write down how you feel after you talk to a particular person or experience a television show, radio program, book, or magazine.

Two Keys in Regaining Control of Your Thoughts

The Worry Break

Take a Worry Break! This is a predetermined amount of time when you do not allow your thoughts to dwell on what is stressing you. First go back over the relaxation skills in the first half of Part II and choose the one that best helps you keep your attention on the present moment. Practice this technique every day to relax and to regain control over your thoughts.

Second, link your mental Worry Break with a daily habit or activity. You may want to take your Worry Break while you jog, shower, commute, do a simple task, or even while you eat a meal. It's your choice. It is easier to replace your worries if you have an activity to focus your attention. Reap the benefit of a Worry Break by consciously holding off worrisome thoughts for a specific length of time or during a specific activity.

The Worry Focus

The Worry Break is particularly effective when coupled with the Worry Focus. Rather than dragging a problem like a ball and chain into all your activities, it is most beneficial to allot a time for both focusing on, and taking a break from, the problem. For half an hour every day, concentrate on a predominant subject of concern—such as an insensitive coworker or boss, the impending layoffs, or a financial predicament. No matter what it is, choose a half hour period to think about it. It can be a time of constructive problem solving, such as listing options, prioritizing, or brainstorming with a coworker. Concentrate fully on what is stressing you.

During the rest of the day, when nagging, stress-filled thoughts reappear on your mental screen, inwardly tell yourself, "No, those thoughts are for the Worry Focus." Discipline your mind. Your Big Worry will retreat because it knows it has its own appointment time with you!

——— USING REFRAMING YOUR
THINKING TECHNIQUES AT WORK ———

Donald came into my office complaining of job stress and marital problems. He slouched dejectedly into his chair, eyes downcast. In a slurred voice he told of his plight. "I can't keep going," he mumbled. "Cindy is talking about taking the kids and leaving. That would kill me. And now, the last straw. With the house mortgaged to the hilt and Jamie needing braces, my supervisor is threatening to fire me. With all my problems at home I can't concentrate at work. I'm making costly mistakes and can't get projects in on time. There is nothing I can do. I worry all the time, can't sleep or even begin to figure out all my problems. Please help me."

Donald's stress due to his troubled marriage was spilling into his work world, resulting in poor productivity and the strain of job insecurity.

We designed a treatment plan partially based on relaxation skills and cognitive exercises. Donald particularly benefited from meditation, and Deep Relaxation with Visualization.

In addition, his wife came in for couples counseling. In the several months it took to get his private life in order, Donald used the Worry Break and Worry Focus techniques at work to help him relax and improve his concentration. Throughout the morning each time his mind turned to his marital problems, he stopped and took three Complete Breaths followed by tensing and relaxing his body three times. This helped bring his focus back to the present and his work. Knowing he would have a Worry Focus time at lunch helped him to keep his worries at bay.

At lunch he took 20 to 30 minutes to focus on how to resolve his marital issues. After his lunch break he used mini-exercise routines and breathing breaks to keep his attention on his work. As he commuted home he used Thought Replacement whenever he caught himself using the thinking distortions of Black and White Thinking or Tunnel Vision regarding his fear of losing his job.

I was most impressed by Donald's success with both the cognitive and relaxation skills. Through diligent practice he was able to minimize his stress. His sleeping patterns improved. His depression lifted and his irritability declined. His concentration at work returned. He lost neither his wife nor his job.

Now use the exercise below to incorporate what you have learned from this chapter into your own work week schedule.

Steps 1 and 2: Write one type of self-talk distortion you habitually make at work and what you will now say to yourself in response:

Old negative talk: _____

_____

New positive talk: _____

_____

Steps 3 and 4: Write one way you can contribute to changing a problem situation or improving your office environment.

Positive step or reinforcement: _____

_____

Worry Break/Worry Focus: Write an example of how you can use the Worry Break/Worry Focus during your work day in combination with a relaxing activity.

My Worry Break will be: _____

_____

My Worry Focus will be:: _____

_____

Changing ingrained negative thought patterns is not something you can achieve overnight. Be patient with yourself. Negative thinking and the negative emotions that accompany it also can distort the way you communicate with others. Learning more positive ways to talk to others at work is the subject of the next chapter.

19

Feelings and Communication
at Work

See people for who they are instead of who you want them to be.
Then accept them as they are rather than judging them for who
they're not.

—Joan Borysenko, *Minding the Body,*
Mending the Mind

How can anyone ever love you for who you are if you become
someone else to be with them?

—Stephen C. Paul, *Illuminations*

Clear communication is the cornerstone to a profitable and positive business atmosphere. Without clear and honest lines of communication, employee happiness, creativity, and productivity suffer.

What is good communication? What styles of communication are useful at work? Should such feelings as anger, depression, or anxiety be expressed in the workplace? If it is appropriate to express feelings on the job, how can you express them in a constructive rather than destructive manner? The answers are as useful at home as on the job.

Good communication clarifies feelings, ideas, or tasks by means of writing, talking, or signaling. When people "mind read," make assumptions not based on fact, or repress feelings, communication may produce more confusion than clarity. Good communication in the workplace is essential for a harmonious work environment as well as for financial success.

In the last chapter you learned how distorted self-talk creates negative emotions, and the importance of reframing your thinking to reduce the intensity of your negative emotions. In this chapter you will learn first, if and when it's appropriate to express emotions at work and how to recognize and defuse emotions before they distort communications. Second, you will learn techniques of assertive communication, ways to ask for what you want and how to set limits in a way that will be productive for you, your supervisor, and your coworkers. Third, you will learn a style of responding to others that acknowledges feelings supportively and "disarms" negativity.

Obstacles to Good Communication at Work

Appropriate and Inappropriate Communications at Work

The issue of communication is sensitive at the worksite, especially when it comes to expressing feelings. Feelings often take a back seat to budgets, deadlines, and productivity. You may not express your feelings at work for a number of reasons. It is your choice not to speak out. It may be a question of selecting which battles to fight. Nevertheless, expression of feelings in the workplace can be appropriate.

At times it may be wiser to hold back or to talk to someone outside of work. If you feel frustrated, you might blow off steam by taking a break, and returning to address the problem without expressing how you feel. You may believe speaking out openly could jeopardize your job. Ultimately, appropriateness is up to you and defined by each situation.

However, clarity in expression, including feelings, can help minimize job stress if it leads to greater understanding and smoother working relationships.

What is typically considered inappropriate, concerns the expression of personal problems and feelings not directly related to the workplace. The following example demonstrates how inappropriate expectations of work relationships can create job stress.

Alice came in for counseling due to job stress. She said, "My boss does not want to hear feelings. He never said a word when I was hospitalized for two weeks due to a car accident on the way to my job. He just wants the job done. I feel used." Alice's anxiety diminished as we explored her conclusion that she was "being used." She came to realize that she did not know why her boss had not made a comment about her accident. Did he keep quiet because a member of his family had been injured in a car accident and it hit too close to his own suffering? Did he feel responsible because she was on her way to work? Did he not want to become involved?

Did he just not know what to say? She had no idea. She could not read his mind. Perhaps Alice cannot expect sympathy from her boss, but she can be honest about her experience with coworkers, and can tell her boss about how the accident affected her. Alice's issue did not revolve around whether or not to express her feelings. Her real issue was her distorted perception regarding her boss's failure to acknowledge her suffering.

This chapter includes exercises designed to help you recognize and integrate the feeling part of yourself into your life. At work, you will need to express this newly emerging side of yourself with discretion. In the following example, Tanya overstepped the bounds of appropriateness.

Tanya, a clerk in a grocery store, began sharing her home problems and personal feelings about company policy with her boss while they were working. After six months of not heeding her boss' suggestions to stay "on task," she was put on probation. In counseling, it became clear that Tanya's self-absorption and negativity were counterproductive. She was hired to do a job, and not be distracted by sharing her feelings. Tanya learned to reframe some of her negativity, take greater interest in her job, and curb her talk regarding domestic problems. Although still on probation, she has learned when and where it is appropriate for her to discuss her feelings.

It is, however, appropriate and necessary to speak up when inappropriate feelings are being directed toward you.

Mona, a legal secretary, quickly and clearly expressed her boundaries when one of the senior partners was inappropriately personal. Because of her firm and clearly stated refusal to comply with him, the lawyer stopped his behavior and avoided further complications.

Although you may believe it is inappropriate to express your feelings in a given work situation, it is helpful to explore your reasoning process. Our thoughts, feelings, and behavior are dictated by our core beliefs. For example, it is easy to surmise the stressful results if Mona had believed it is *never* appropriate to express her boundaries to a boss. Core beliefs govern our interpretation of ourselves and the world around us. Just as a gardener must dig out the roots to prevent future regrowth of a weed, so must we unearth hidden beliefs which control how we think and feel, and thus communicate. If we can discover what our core beliefs are, we can decide whether they are useful or limiting in our current situation (McKay and Fanning, 1992).

Discomfort with Feelings

Many people are uncomfortable with their feelings or afraid of the reaction of others. Their confusion around feelings is a stumbling block to honest, open relationships at work. Dorothy provides a good example.

Dorothy, a clerk in a large department store, did not feel it was appropriate to express her anger to her supervisor. She had asked the store manager several times if he would run interference for her. Although he agreed to do so, he never followed through on his promises. In counseling, Dorothy and I explored her reluctance to speak directly to her supervisor. I asked, "What emotions are you afraid to express to your supervisor?" "Anger," she replied. "Why?" "She will reject me." "What if she does reject you, what does that mean to you?" "That she doesn't like me." "What if she doesn't like you, what does that mean to you?" "It means that I am an unworthy person." This dialogue brought to light that Dorothy's fear of expressing anger was based on her lack of self-esteem (McKay and Fanning, 1992). After further exploration and clarification of other feelings masked by her anger, and some self-esteem work, Dorothy spoke to her supervisor. The supervisor appreciated the discussion and it led the way to a much warmer, productive working relationship.

Are you confused or uneasy about your feelings or those of a coworker? Do you avoid emotions by directing the conversation to tasks or ideas? If so, you are maneuvering away from your discomfort by analyzing away the emotional atmosphere. When life is hurtful, one solution is to escape from a feeling mode into a thinking mode. To cope with a painful or confusing environment, some people shut down or become numb to their feelings. This maneuver is usually developed in childhood to protect oneself from emotional pain. Most likely it was a suitable and healthy response for a child to maintain sanity. Later in life it may be safe and beneficial for your self-esteem to expand the feeling side of yourself. Like using an atrophied muscle, it takes time and practice to become comfortable with your own emotions.

Do you deny you are having a problem at work? Do you consider it a sign of weakness to admit to being anxious, angry, or overwhelmed when stretched to the breaking point? Or do you assume that your feelings are obvious and coworkers should know what you are feeling? Even though you feel hurt, exhausted, or resentful, do you avoid expressing your feelings because you believe others' needs are more important than yours? Do you ignore your needs and feelings to meet others' needs, no matter what the cost?

Even though well-intentioned, these flawed styles—making diversionary tactics and analyzing maneuvers (to avoid expressing emotions), denying feelings, making accommodating gestures, giving double messages (saying one thing but indicating something else by tone or gesture)—all indicate the difficulty we have with expression of our own or others' feelings, and muddy rather than clarify communication. They are often based on false beliefs or low self-esteem. The more we have confidence in ourselves, the easier it is to be open and honest. These styles imply that you do not honor yourself.

Improving your ability to recognize and express your feelings will expand your options, deepen your self-understanding, and improve your self-esteem.

Lack of Communication Skills

The exercises below will help you to learn more about your emotions: how to identify and manage them. Once you are comfortable with your feelings, you will be able to more easily communicate your needs, limits, frustrations, and concerns to coworkers and management.

If you are uncertain about how to initiate your discussion and what to say, a section follows that will define using non-defensive "I-messages" and "scripting" your communication in advance.

Expanding Awareness and Expression of Feelings

The following exercises will help you to gain trust and confidence in your feelings, and the ability to express them appropriately at work if and when you choose to do so. They are designed to help those who are uncomfortable expressing their feelings. They will help you express yourself from the heart in a way that is desirable. The exercises are graduated to allow you to gain confidence as you practice. The goal is to have *both* the thinking and feeling aspects of yourself at your disposal.

One mistaken belief is that confrontation will be avoided if you don't express your feelings or if you accommodate to the inappropriate behavior of others. This approach either leads to depression, or creates an underlying tension that will emerge more intensely at a later date. Let's look at how to reduce stress by learning how to recognize and express or release work-related depression, anger, and anxiety.

STEPS TO REDUCE WORK-RELATED DEPRESSION, ANGER, AND ANXIETY

There are three steps in reducing work-related depression, anger and anxiety.

Step 1.: Recognizing body cues that express feelings. For example, identifying a tightness in the chest as an expression of worry, or sagging posture and sighing might be expressions of depression, or a tight jaw an expression of pent-up anger. Body awareness gives you information about what you are feeling.

Step 2. Identifying feelings in their early stage. Learn what you are feeling before it becomes an intense or overwhelming emotion. For example, recognizing your uneasiness before it becomes fear, or your frustration before it becomes rage.

Step 3: Reducing the intensity of an emotion. Learn to release or express it before it distorts communication.

   a. Indirect options: Release intensity through such coping skills as relaxation breaks, exercise, or writing.

   b. Direct options: Express yourself using assertive communication and good listening skills.

Preparing for Step 1: Monitoring Your Body's Responses

Neutral and Positive Experiences

For a safe beginning to reestablishing an awareness of your feelings, experience moments of relaxation, wonder, or joy which you have overlooked, and then become aware of your body. Have you ever eaten a meal and then realized you never really tasted it? With the fast paced lives we are leading, we do not enjoy what is right in front of us. Our busy minds keep us from the present moment. Quiet your mind enough to enjoy the now. Your burdens won't disappear, but you will be better prepared to handle them.

For one week, while doing menial tasks or relaxing, ask yourself how your body is responding to the present experience. Rather than mentally organize your morning's schedule during a shower, note how the warm water feels on your shoulders. And enjoy it! How does the sun feel on your face as you walk from your car to the office? Does it feel good to stretch your legs as you get out of the car? Monitor your body when you are enjoying an interesting novel or relaxing in front of the fire. Does your jaw relax, or your headache diminish? Notice how your body responds when you awaken to various neutral and positive sensations throughout the day. Record your experiences below.

Neutral/Positive Experience   *Physical Response/Behavioral Cue*

_____   _____

_____   _____

_____   _____

_____   _____

_____   _____

_____   _____

_____   _____

_____   _____

_____   _____

_____   _____

Negative Experiences

Once you are in the habit of being aware of your physical responses to neutral and positive moments, expand your attention to include responses to negative experiences. Do you get a headache or queasy stomach when a coworker asks you to finish his assignment? When the noise level increases at the office do you find yourself clenching your jaw? What work situations trigger physical discomfort? Are your negative physical responses triggered by the work environment, your relationships at work, or the work itself? Link your physical responses to specific circumstances and record your observations below. When you increase your awareness of subtle body signals you will simultaneously increase your awareness of your frame of mind.

Negative Experience   *Physical Response/Behavioral Cue*

_____   _____

_____   _____

_____   _____

_____   _____

_____   _____

_____   _____

_____   _____

_____   _____

_____   _____

Now use the awareness you've gained doing these exercises to monitor the physical cues that indicate you are becoming depressed, angry, or anxious. The following exercises will ask you to identify these physical cues, then add Steps 2 and 3, identifying the feelings and reducing their intensity.

Depression at Work: Recognizing Your Boundaries

If you do not express your needs and feelings in order to "keep the peace" at work or home, the result can be depression. Have you lost your sense of identity? Do you feel empty and confused? Have you stopped expressing your hopes and goals at work out of fear of rejection, demotion, or ridicule? If you consistently hold back your feelings and needs, you gradually lose touch with what you feel or need. If you are denying yourself, you lose yourself, and when you lose yourself, you become depressed.

Recognizing Your Stages of Depression

Below is a list of feelings that progressively lead up to depression. It is vital to identify and monitor your feelings leading up to depression so that you can act on and release these feelings before you become overwhelmed.

Quiet
Sad
Declining enthusiasm
Reduced energy
Lonely
Withdrawn
Melancholy
Sense of helplessness
Feeling overwhelmed

Use the chart below to list what you feel are your stages of depression and your corresponding physical or behavioral response to each one.

Stages of Depression   *Physical Responses/Behavioral Cues*

_____   _____

_____   _____

_____   _____

_____   _____

_____   _____

_____   _____

_____   _____

_____   _____

Reducing the Intensity of Your Depression

To prevent yourself from continuing in a downward spiral toward helplessness and being overwhelmed, take steps to lighten your load. Remember, you become depressed when you lose touch with yourself: your own feelings and needs. Before you become depressed, choose a stress-reducing tool that is just for you. The following are some suggestions.

☐ Say "no" to certain activities and people

☐ Pamper yourself; give yourself a gift

☐ Replace negative self-talk about yourself with positive affirmations

☐ Take a brisk walk, preferably in nature

☐ Avoid overload; prioritize

☐ Reduce sugar, fat, and caffeine

☐ Use Creative Time activities

☐ Ask for help; delegate workload

Use the following chart to record situations at work where you began to experience the beginning stages of depression. Add to this chart steps you could take to reduce and release these feelings.

Work Stressor	Stage of Depression	Physical/Behavioral Cue	Stress-Reducing Response
_____	_____	_____	_____
_____	_____	_____	_____
_____	_____	_____	_____
_____	_____	_____	_____
_____	_____	_____	_____

The direct approach, speaking out, may be the best solution to alleviate your depression. If you need help with this, see the section on assertive communication.

Anger at Work: Preventing Escalation

Rather than feeling depressed, do you stuff your emotions until they explode like an erupting volcano? If you have shut down the feeling side of yourself, you might ask, "What emotions do I experience? Is anger one of them?" Do you talk with excessive intensity, wave your arms, angrily blame or shout, or pound a table? Offensive displays of anger can be prevented by recognizing and expressing feelings before they accumulate and intensify.

The following exercises will help you become aware of feelings leading up to anger, and how to express them appropriately. This will prevent a build-up of tension. By learning to recognize your own stages of anger, you will also more readily discern them in others, which will enable you to get clarification before their emotions peak.

Recognizing Your Stages of Anger

Many people may be unaware they are angry until they explode in a rage. If you try to communicate your anger when it is overwhelming you, others will feel overwhelmed, too, and may shut out what you legitimately want to express. Below is a sample list of feelings that progressively lead up to rage. It is important to learn to monitor your own experience of anger so you can release it and/or express it at an earlier stage.

Uneasy

Uncomfortable

Irritated

Annoyed

Perturbed

Upset

Frustrated

Mad

Angry

Furious

Enraged

Use the chart below to list what you feel are your stages of anger. To help, turn your attention to your physical response to each one. Do you clench your fists or tense your shoulders when you are irritated? Do you notice your breathing pattern change or your stomach tense when you are upset? Write your physical response next to each escalating feeling of anger. These body signals can help you recognize what stage of anger you are experiencing.

Stages of Anger   *Physical Responses/Behavioral Cues*

_____   _____

_____   _____

_____   _____

_____   _____

_____   _____

_____   _____

Becoming familiar with your feelings and physical responses that lead up to rage can give you a sense of control. Then you can choose what would be the appropriate expression of these feelings. There are appropriate means of expressing and releasing tension before reaching rage. You need not wait for the familiar moment of crisis. However, before you decide to express your anger, you may want to find out if anger is all you are feeling.

Reducing the Intensity of Your Anger

As you get better at recognizing your feelings and expressing them, you will begin to notice that what you labeled as one emotion may be just the surface layer disguising other emotions. For example, an angry feeling can be a mask for feeling hurt, attacked, betrayed, or fearful. As you come to understand your feelings, you can appropriately communicate these feelings, or resolve the issues causing the feelings. Sometimes it's difficult to appreciate the complexity of your emotions about a person or situation. The following exercise can be used whenever you need clarification. This process is effective in reducing feelings of anger. Use it as a response to work situations in which you feel yourself escalating toward rage.

The Circle Exercise. Draw a circle on a plain sheet of paper. Next to it list the primary emotions you have toward a person or situation. Using colored pens, make pie pieces that express the intensity or amount of that feeling. The act of drawing the feelings helps crystalize what emotions you are experiencing. Draw the circle weekly. Your emotions may remain unchanged over a period of time, or you may uncover unexpected feelings. Just let whatever feelings you have come up. Below is a black and white example of a client's growing understanding of his feelings regarding a coworker.

> *Allan came to counseling in a rage—the only emotion he was aware of feeling. He drew the circle exercise over a three week period. Notice that at first he thought he was primarily angry. Over the weeks he realized some of the emotions hidden beneath his anger. Once he had a clearer sense of the complexity of his feelings, he worked on those related to his own lack of self-esteem—guilt, embarrassment, and hurt. Once he had taken responsibility for his share of the problem, his anger was less intense and he could communicate it in a calm yet firm manner.*

To further reduce and manage your anger, find appropriate ways of expressing your stages of anger. The following are lists of some inappropriate and appropriate responses. Check off ones you currently use.

Inappropriate Responses	**Appropriate Responses**
☐ Yell/Scream	☐ State: I feel ____.
☐ Talk harshly	☐ Go for a jog
☐ Hit/Throw objects	☐ Time-Out—Leave, talk later
☐ Mull/Stew/Fume	☐ Do a relaxation exercise
☐ Withdraw, Clam up	☐ Listen, ask questions
☐ Eat/drink/smoke—to cover up feelings	☐ Write out feelings

Allan's Feelings Regarding Fellow Worker

First Circle—Week One

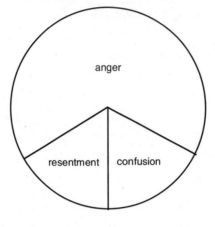

Second Circle—Week Two

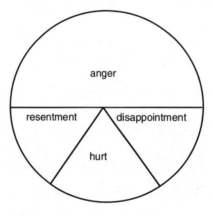

Third Circle—Week Three

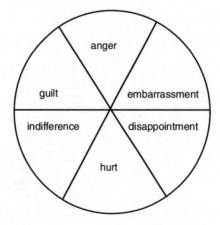

☐ Blame self or blame others

☐ Complain loudly to coworkers

☐ Take it out on people at home

☐ Assertively express needs

☐ Talk at a support group

☐ Problem-solve

☐ Seek counseling to resolve past conflict

As you seek to choose more appropriate ways to express your anger, you may find your intensity is rooted in your past. Are current problems an outgrowth of unresolved past conflict? For example, does an angry boss remind you of a critical parent? If you answered "Yes!" to these questions, resolution of your anger involves sorting out your feelings regarding past issues. If your job tension is aggravated because of unsolved personal pain, defuse your anger through counseling, or by attending a support group.

Anger management always concludes with problem solving. Self-understanding, open communication, compromise, and attention to solutions eliminate current anger. The direct approach to relieving anger is to resolve the conflict which caused the anger. In the section on assertive communication you will learn skills to help you if you decide to voice your irritation.

Reducing Anxiety at Work: Managing Your Fears

Anxiety, like depression and anger, is an emotion that many people ignore or cannot identify in its earlier stages. Anxiety becomes more intense as unease magnifies into fear. The probability of a positive outcome diminishes as one's attention dwells on negative possibilities. Action is paralyzed in a quagmire of doubt or squandered in scattered, desultory planning.

You can take charge of your anxiety and release your stress by first learning to recognize the level of stress you are experiencing. Your body's distress signals reveal your level of tension. Use this awareness to identify the feelings behind your increasing tension.

Recognizing Your Stages of Anxiety

Below is a list of feelings that lead up to anxiety. It is important to take steps to reduce your distress and relax before you start to feel panicked.

Disquieted

Impatient

Edgy

Concerned

Wary, Apprehensive

Worried

Nervous

Fearful

Distressed

Alarmed

Panicked

Use the chart below to list what you feel are your stages of anxiety and your corresponding physical or behavioral cues to each one.

Stages of Anxiety   *Physical Responses/Behavioral Cues*

_____   _____

_____   _____

_____   _____

_____   _____

_____   _____

Reducing the Intensity of Your Anxiety

Take steps to reduce your level of tension before it magnifies into increased anxiety. Below is a brief list of indirect ways you can release your tension and calm yourself.

☐ Deep, Conscious Breathing

☐ Nature Visualization

☐ Deep Relaxation

☐ Gentle Stretching

☐ Quiet Time alone

☐ Worry Breaks

☐ Prioritize your workload

☐ Walk, preferably outside

☐ Drink tea; cut down or eliminate caffeine

On the following chart, record experiences you have recently had at work when you felt increasing anxiety and tension. In the last column, choose a stress-reducing response that you would use to soothe yourself. Use the list above, other skills from the previous chapters, or methods that have worked for you in the past.

Work Stressor	Level of Anxiety	Physical/Behavioral Cues	Stress-Reducing Response
_____	_____	_____	_____
_____	_____	_____	_____
_____	_____	_____	_____
_____	_____	_____	_____
_____	_____	_____	_____
_____	_____	_____	_____
_____	_____	_____	_____

If you decide to express your concerns directly, turn to the next section on assertive communication for ways to appropriately and safely voice your worries.

Assertive Communication

Assertive communication is expressing yourself—your needs, feelings, and perspective—in a manner which is clear, direct, and neither threatening nor attacking. Learning a specific structure for communicating can reduce your stress and confusion about how to address a coworker or management regarding a difficult situation.

In this section you will be given tips on assertive communications that include scripting (writing or practicing) what you want to say in what are called I-messages. I-messages have three parts: I think, I feel, I want. The "I think" is your objective description of the facts or problem. The "I feel" acknowledges your reaction without blaming or trying to intimidate. The "I want" part is your request for a change or for more information. I-messages improve productivity and harmony at work by dealing directly with a stressful situation, without blaming or criticizing. Rather than pointing the finger with a blaming you-statement, you clarify your understanding, needs, or feelings with I-statements to prevent escalation of emotions.

Assertive communication as a stress management tool means expressing your feelings and opinions openly, especially *before* you are overwhelmed. Once you are aware of your body's responses to positive and negative situations, *begin* to express yourself more openly. Start with the easy ones—neutral or positive I-statements—such as a simple "I feel great. This is a project I can really sink my teeth into. Thanks!" Use your experience of monitoring body responses to help you know what you are feeling.

Once you are comfortable with neutral or positive statements, begin to express harder ones such as, "I feel annoyed when you don't look at me while I am speaking." No longer ignore your anger or other negative feelings. If appropriate, voice your concerns. These personal skills lead to a broader, more relaxed, expressive you at work. It does not mean you become a touchy-feely person, but it does mean that you become a person who is congruent; one who can, when relevant, honestly express what is going on internally.

If speaking out would jeopardize your job, then compromise. Express your feelings to a friend, a therapist, or your spouse. Get the feelings out, but not where it would do you harm. Now let's look at how to express the feelings behind depression, anger, and anxiety. This section will give you added information on how to express your feelings assertively.

Assertive communication is based on specific assumptions. Basic ones are:

1. Your feelings are legitimate.

2. You have the right to ask questions.

3. It's O.K. to negotiate for change.

4. It is your right to set boundaries, to say "no."

5. You know better than anyone what you think, feel, or need (Davis et al., 1988).

If you are depressed, angry, or anxious, and want to express yourself directly, keep these assumptions in mind to bolster your self-confidence.

To develop a sense of well-being and fulfillment, it is necessary to express and act on inner needs. Honor your needs. Don't sacrifice who you are for the good of all. Understand your limits and set clear boundaries. This allows the people around you to adjust accordingly. You are part of a whole, and as important as any member of the group. The solution lies in compromise, but not a compromise of ideals and needs. If all members of a group express their ideals and needs, the differences will be apparent, and solutions to problems can then incorporate the ideals and needs of each member.

You may be depressed because you are allowing people at work to manipulate you. Rather than setting limits by expressing your needs, are you taking on extra assignments, staying late, or doing others' projects for them? Instead of blaming them for your exhaustion, set clear boundaries by saying, "No."

Consider your possible beliefs that let others take advantage of you at work:

1. The needs of others are more important than mine.

2. To be liked or approved of, I must "be there" for others, no matter what my emotional or physical cost.

3. It would be selfish of me to put my needs first.

If any of the above apply to you, an important factor in your depression is low self-esteem. Communicate your needs. Don't think that people value you or like you more if they can control you. To be used is not to be respected or liked. Allowing yourself to be used only reinforces your negative view of yourself and intensifies your depression. Obviously, you want to lend a helping hand when others are in need, but when you feel annoyance, anger, or resentment, respond to these signals. They are informing you of your boundaries. As appropriate to the situation, voice your feelings using I-messages. Verbalizing your feelings improves communication and self-esteem.

As with depression, it can be appropriate to express your anger and anxiety at work. If irritation or worries remain unvoiced, misunderstandings become magnified. People cannot respond correctly if they do not know what you are experiencing. After you have examined and defused your anger and anxiety you will find you can communicate with clarity by using I-messages. Being able to express your anger assertively in its early stages, without blame, avoids putting the other person on the defensive.

Express your anxiety in its earlier stages. If you are doubtful about a project, voice your concern to a supervisor. Don't wait until you are alarmed by a situation. Consult with a coworker. Reveal your worries at a staff meeting, especially if you have constructive alternatives. Do your homework first. Express your uncertainty in the form of options, not right and wrong. If you back up your position with facts and figures, others can respond appropriately whether it be corroboration, a supportive ear, or other options.

If you find that it is not to your best interests to voice your fears, talk with someone outside the office setting. It's important to have support. Do not isolate yourself by mentally withdrawing into a critical or increasingly anxious mode. Being alone with your troubles makes them more threatening to you. The final section on Using Good Communication at Work will give you an example and exercise to practice scripting and I-messages for resolving a stressful work situation.

Good Listening Skills

In addition to expressing yourself through I-messages, work site stress can be reduced by using good listening skills. Everyone wants to be heard and supported whether male or female, supervisor or coworker. The following components of good listening—being attentive, disarming, and supportive—aid in improving interpersonal relationships at work.

The Attentive Listener. One of the best ways to reduce communication-related stress is to be a good listener. Lack of clarity causes misunderstanding. Do not concentrate on your response while the other person is talking. If necessary, jot down a word or two as reminders, but do your best to *be attentive* to the words, tone, and body language of the other person. Often there are double messages. What is being said may not be congruent with gestures or tone, and you need to be aware of this duality to understand better.

When another person has finished speaking, one of the best responses is to *mirror back* what you think has been conveyed. Paraphrase what was said. "Are you saying that. . .?" "If I understand you correctly, . . . " Stay with that part of the conversation until the other person has finished, and until it is clear to you what they have said. Do not assume too much. Do not try to mind read. If you are confused, clarify by questioning, using the mirroring style. You might say, "I'm not sure if you mean _____ or _____ ."

If a feeling comes up in response to another person's statements, an attentive listener might let the other person know how the statement affected him. Without blaming, you simply say, "When you do or say_____ , I feel _____ , because _____ ." This prevents an escalation of accusations. You are not blaming, you are giving information. At this point, the attentive listener becomes the assertive communicator.

The Disarmer. How do you react to criticism? When uncomfortable with disapproval from a coworker or supervisor, do you make a joke or change the subject as a diversionary tactic? Or does your embarrassment or inability to admit your error lead you to not respond or blame someone or something else? If you are innocent, how do you defend yourself?

It is not easy to admit fault. It is especially difficult if admitting an error leads to self-recrimination and feelings of guilt. The best way to grow out of this pattern is to listen to the criticism openly, and to disarm the other person by saying, "Yes, you have a point there. I'll explore it." Then analyze the criticism for any truth. Look at the possibility that they are right. Use the information to better yourself or the project. Perfectionism is a trap. You are O.K., even if you make a mistake. In fact, people almost always respect the person who can admit a mistake. People recognize that taking responsibility for an error requires confidence and courage. Clowning around at a staff meeting when criticized, or changing the subject when at fault is obvious to everyone and helpful to nobody.

If possible, separate *how* a person expresses themselves from *what* they are saying. For example, if your boss uses an exasperated tone, exaggerates, or even belittles you, ignore the negative style and listen to the information.

Agree only to the truth of what is said. If a statement is untrue or reflects someone's perceptions or doubts projected onto you, respond by saying something like, "Yes, I understand what you are saying, but I do not agree."

How do you criticize others? If you need to point out someone else's error, do it in the disarming style. Point out their errors in a nonjudgmental tone, with facts and figures, and allow that person room to express his or her side of a situation. Don't say, "You've blown it for the fourth time this week, Sam. Get your act together, or you're out." Instead, you might say, "I have checked, there is no glitch on Judy's computer program. It's your errors on assignment of orders that are creating incorrect mailings at the warehouse. This cannot continue. What's the problem? What do you recommend?"

Another method is to sandwich the critique between two true and positive statements. This makes criticism more palatable to the listener. For example, if a project is turned in late or has errors, first communicate what you appreciate about the job, then point out the problem, and close with another reassurance.

The Supporter. Imagine a coworker saying to you, "I've run into an incredible glitch on the Hammerstein case. I've discovered a conflict of interest for our firm. Jake is out of town but he asked me to send these papers to the opposing attorney this afternoon. I am in a quandary as to what to do." After a bit more input, the coworker turns to you for a response. What do you say? There are two basic approaches: a) give suggestions that would solve his dilemma or b) be supportive and sympathetic with the problem he is facing. Which do you normally do, give solutions first or give support first?

> *Sandra and Aaron came into my office on the verge of divorce. They owned and operated a small construction firm in which she was the accountant. Due to a depression in the housing market, construction was almost at a standstill. Their business was on the brink of bankruptcy. When she approached him in a quandary on how to stretch out payment of overdue bills, he would withdraw to his office without comment. She responded with hurt and anger.*
>
> *Further discussion revealed that Aaron thought Sandy expected him to have solutions to the financial issues she raised. Because he was embarrassed that he did not know how to solve their problems, he would withdraw. This information surprised Sandy. What she had wanted was support. She knew there was no easy answer to their financial straits. She just needed him to listen and talk about the difficult situation. This revelation for both of them cleared the air and led to other points of miscommunication. In only three sessions they realized it was not the issues that were driving them apart, but their miscommunication.*

Since childhood women have been trained to be empathic. Women are usually comfortable with feelings and respond naturally with understanding and sympathy. On the other hand, men, since childhood, have been trained to seek solutions to any given problem. They tend to be action-oriented rather than feeling-oriented. In recent years this has become less a gender issue, but it is still important to be aware of the problems inherent in a conversation between a feeling-oriented person and an action-oriented person. They may arrive at the same conclusion, but the process and emphasis are different. If you are having problems communicating with your supervisor or a coworker, be aware of this difference. Indicate with an I-message that you wish to listen and talk supportively about the situation rather than receive or provide specific solutions.

USING GOOD COMMUNICATION AT WORK

If you plan to speak directly to a coworker or manager regarding a situation that is causing you stress, it is helpful to clearly identify through scripting the problem, your feelings, and what you are going to say in the form of I-statements. Also keep in mind that you will want to be a good listener by listening attentively, disarming criticism if necessary, and being supportive of the other person's views and feelings. Below is Jan's example of how scripting helped her approach her boss.

Jan's Situation
The boss is overloading me with work again, and he's always giving me extra work late in the afternoon when I'm tired. Yet he expects me to rush the job and get it done by 5 p.m.

Jan's Feelings

I'm mad. I'm fed up. I'm feeling taken advantage of, but I'm afraid to talk to him. I'm afraid he'll blame me.

Indirect Expression

I'll take a walk and Worry Break at lunch to relax. I'll write about my feelings in my journal.

Direct Expression

When I get back from lunch I'll ask to talk to him before the afternoon pile appears on my desk.

Jan's Script

Using the three-part I-messages:

I think: Recently you have been giving me work late in the day and expecting it to be done by 5 p.m.

I feel: I feel overwhelmed and anxious about getting it all done. I feel rushed and pressured and less productive.

I want: If you have an important project, I would like to know about it early in the morning so I can plan my day. I would like to get such projects before lunch whenever possible.

Jan's boss apologized to her for overloading her with work. He admitted he was disorganized, which led to rushing at the end of the day. He agreed to discuss the workload in the morning and to prioritize and coordinate their schedules. This led to regular morning meetings that prepared them both for the day.

Use the exercise below to help you resolve a stressful situation at work.

Situation: _____

_____

Feelings: _____

_____

Indirect Expression (Reduce Intensity of Feelings): _____

_____

Direct Expression (Communicate Assertively):

I think: _____

_____

I feel: _____

_____

I want: _____

_____

Part of your stress could be related to a lack of communication at home. Apply these techniques to communications at home and you will be less stressed at work as a result. As best you can, apply them at work, along with the stress management skills you have learned.

The next chapter, on ways to expand your social support network, can also help you if you are having difficulties with your feelings and communicating assertively. Perhaps you can practice your assertiveness "script" with someone in your social support network before you talk to your supervisor or a coworker.

20

Social Support: The Best Medicine

*Illness, a shorter life expectancy, and less satisfaction in life are
likely companions to those individuals who fail to master the
opportunities and responsibilities of friendships.*

—J.M. Witmer and T.J. Sweeney, *A Holistic Model
for Wellness and Prevention Over the Life Span*

A friend is a present you give yourself.

—Robert Louis Stevenson

The single most important ingredient in your recipe for wellness is a strong social support system. A wealth of new research shows that loving, caring relationships enhance your mental and physical well-being.

- People with friends are less likely to suffer from physical and mental ill health than those who are socially isolated (California Department of Mental Health, 1981).

- A recent study of 7,000 people over a nine year period revealed people with few ties to others had two to five times the death rate as those who had more ties (Witmer and Sweeney, 1992).

- The same study also found that connection with other people was more important to maintaining health than smoking, drinking, exercise, or diet.

- Loneliness is statistically associated with depression, suicide, alcohol abuse, anxiety, poor self-esteem, decreased activity of the immune system, and increased mortality (Witmer and Sweeney, 1992).

What is social support? It is the evidence that someone out there cares for you and, in return, that you are concerned about others. It is active participation in the circle of giving and receiving. Social support is made up of three components:

- emotional support—being able to confide in or rely on another.

- tangible support—direct help, such as loans, gifts, or helping out (for example, bringing a snack to a coworker who is under pressure to meet a deadline).

- informational support—providing information, advice, or feedback (California Department of Mental Health, 1981).

There is a direct correlation between this "social connectedness" and depression, anxiety, and a host of physical diseases. We need social support most acutely during times of physical or emotional crisis—when we experience an overload of stressors. The need is the same regardless of whether there is too much stimulation or too little, or whether the stress arises out of a positive circumstance such as a promotion or a negative one such as a layoff.

Family, friends, or other social support help protect us from the harmful effects of stress. According to etiological studies, there has been a dramatic breakdown in the traditional family and community infrastructure in the last 60 to 70 years. The roots of social cohesion are being severed by the constant mobility of the population. Extended families are now typically fractured into separate, isolated units, often at great distance from each other. Immediate families live alone in suburbs and cities without the traditional support of aunts, uncles, cousins, grandparents, and generations of family friends. This deterioration of family connections has also weakened the community support system, so that in times of a community crisis such as an earthquake or power outage we often observe looting and violence in the aftermath rather than help and support.

The pervasive sense of being strangers in an alien society demands that we make a concerted effort to create new avenues for community caring.

How to Get the Support You Need

Within the first two counseling sessions, I always ask my clients: "What are your support systems? Who is there for you? Do you have a close relationship with family members? Do they live nearby? Do you have friends at work? Do you socialize during coffee and lunch breaks? Do you belong to a church or social group?" Learning how to create a sense of belonging, of being part of a social system, greatly enriches the life of the client.

My treatment plan always includes discussion of ways and means to reestablish relationships or build new ones. I am not alone in using social support as a part of treatment. It is an integral part of psychotherapy. For example, as a clinical administrator for a large insurance company, I conduct "utilization reviews"—interviews with therapists who are seeking authorization for additional sessions with their clients—and the condition of the client's support system is one of the six areas I am required to review.

Whether your stress is due to a situation at work or at home, a support system is valuable. The following are suggestions for creating or reestablishing a network of support.

In the Workplace

- Connect with coworkers. It is healthy to connect with at least one or two coworkers on a personal level. This does not necessarily mean socializing beyond the job site, but rather sharing a coffee break, having lunch, or taking walks with a fellow worker, or sharing a personal event such as a son's promotion or a daughter's first date. Briefly asking about someone's health or offering a supportive ear if they look troubled creates a warmer, happier workplace.

- Management's role. Management can play a major role in creating a support system by making sure every worker is part of a network. For example, secretaries are often left out of business meetings and have no organized group format of their own. They feel left out of the decision-making process, isolated from the goals of the company and not valued for their experience and knowledge. This does not mean every employee needs to be at every meeting; rather, that every employee is more productive and happier when included in some form of group process. The important role of managers in creating a supportive workplace is discussed in more detail in Part IV.

If you are not in management, use your new assertive communication skills to call for a meeting with management to discuss ways to create a wellness-focused workplace or ways to enhance a teamwork atmosphere.

- Take a class. An informal way to connect with people while learning a new skill, hobby, or physical discipline is to take a class. There may be classes available through work or work-related classes, perhaps even paid for by your company. Check your local college or high school for adult education classes or your local newspaper for private classes.

- Use on-site employee programs. Take advantage of employee on-site wellness programs. Take an on-site aerobics class with a coworker. Look into other ways the company provides services for employees and explore what is offered.

- Consider volunteer work. Volunteering helps build a sense of community—of being willing to make other people's problems your own so that you can solve them together. Helping others takes you beyond your problems and improves self-esteem. Do something about a problem and you will find yourself empowered, relieved of a sense of hopelessness. You *do* make a difference! In addition, through volunteer work you meet other volunteers as well as those you are serving.

  At work there may be volunteer programs or fund drives you can support. Is there an activity you can organize such as a volleyball team, a picnic, or doing something for a coworker who is ill?

- Join a group that inspires you. Inspiration comes in all forms. What organization or group might help you feel supported? Is it your church? Or is there a nature awareness society, hiking club, or poetry reading group you would like to join? There may be a club that expands on your work interests. Ask people at work if they know of interesting or fun groups.

- Purchase a plant. Beautify your office with flowers or a plant. Even a small gesture like this connects you with life around you. Taking care of a plant and watching it grow and blossom helps to bond you with nature. This could be a first small step towards ecological awareness and concern. Whether you recycle newspapers or compost organic waste, you experience an increased sense of planetary connectedness. It helps break your sense of isolation.

Outside the Workplace

- Call a friend or family member. Ask if they have time to listen. Often, in these busy times, people can share and "be there" for you by telephone, even if they cannot see you personally. Calling them when you are stressed also allows them to send you a card or to call back later. Too often people do not know that a friend is in crisis, saying afterward, "If only I had known." Let them be there for you.

- Take time to laugh. Friendship means relaxation, enjoyment, and laughter. Positive emotions in general have a salutary effect on your well-being. An excellent stress reducer!

- Join a support group. Whether your issues are around childhood trauma or current addictions, there are numerous AA-type support groups. There are "Tough Love" groups for parents having severe problems managing "incorrigible" children. There are support groups for depression and grief, and numerous other issues. Check with your doctor, call your local hospital for information, call your local mental health department, or look in the Yellow Pages.

- Consider obtaining a pet. What joys an animal friend can bring you. My cat, Woody, has certainly enriched my life! Animals are playful, nonjudgmental, and a wonderful source of companionship and joy.

Connecting with coworkers, your community, family, friends, animals, or nature is good medicine!

———— *USING SOCIAL SUPPORT AT WORK* ————

If you are stressed at work because you feel isolated or left out, look over the suggestions above and come up with some of your own to create a list of four ways you can increase your sense of feeling supported and connected to others while at work (or at home).

Ways I can increase my social support at work.

1. _____

2. _____

3. _____

4. _____

The next chapter is especially relevant to today's working woman, who often needs extra support as she attempts to balance the demands of career and family life. This will be followed by the chapter that gives you the opportunity to compile the skills and choices you've made in the preceding chapters into your Wellness Program.

21

Especially for Working Women

*In order to heal our bodies, we have to reenter them and
experience them. Be open to the messages and mysteries of your
body and its symptoms. Be eager to listen and slow to judge.
What you learn may have the capacity to save your life.*

—Christiane Northrup,
Women's Bodies, Women's Wisdom

Women becoming a significant part of the work force not only has economic and social impact but health implications too. Women are particularly vulnerable to stress as their social roles evolve to include work as well as the traditional roles of wife and mother.

It is a career, not necessarily marriage, that glimmers in the eye of the young woman graduating from high school or college. The rewards of economic independence and intellectual and creative stimulation beckon. Two-income families have become the norm. Almost two-thirds of the women in the work force have children under 18 years of age, and 53 percent of the women in the work force have children under six years old (International Labor Office, 1993).

These women face the rigors of a career and the demands of a family. Men are increasingly partners in home front duties, but women continue to do 70 percent of household chores and childrearing tasks. A working mother faces job-related projects, deadlines, and interpersonal pressures along with family responsibilities such as doing the grocery shopping and laundry, and arranging child care, car pooling, music lessons, and doctor appointments. This can be a logistical nightmare. What can she do when Johnny gets sick? What are her alternatives when the baseball team changes its schedule to Thursdays—the one day the sitter has other plans? Is this the final straw that turns a mom's hard work, enthusiasm, and ambition into overwhelm and frustration? Women are under more stress than ever before!

Joining the work force also suggests an increasingly sedentary life style. Working usually implies minimal physical activity. It entails sitting in cars, subways, buses, trains, limousines, taxis, and airplanes. It means standing in elevators, sitting at desks or computer terminals, and sitting still more at business lunches. These sedentary activities replace the more active home life of house cleaning, picking up and chasing after the children, and running errands.

The sedentary life style, on top of enormous social expectations, is showing up as increased stress-related physical and mental illnesses for women.

- On average, one in two women will develop cardiovascular illness. Cardiovascular illness statistics no longer apply solely to men: women have heart attacks, strokes, and high blood pressure. An inactive, sedentary life style almost doubles the risk of coronary heart disease (Cooper, 1978).

- On average, one American woman in eight will contract breast cancer at some point in her life.

- One woman in three will contract osteoporosis (Korn, 1994).

- Women are also facing such stress-related illnesses as anxiety attacks, depression, insomnia, and migraine headaches.

Four of the leading causes of death in America are related to life style: poor eating, lack of exercise, smoking, and drinking (Korn, 1994). Healthy eating, regular exercise, quitting smoking, and reducing alcohol intake significantly reduces your chances of developing heart disease, lung and breast cancer, strokes, diabetes (Type II—adult onset), or osteoporosis.

The stressful and sedentary life style associated with work is costly to your health and happiness only if you don't do something about it. We can keep our lives in balance through setting boundaries and allowing time for self-care. You can reduce your chance of suffering from physical and mental illnesses through life style choices. You can reduce health risks and dramatically improve your quality of life if you choose to exercise, eat nutritious foods, and take time for you.

Being a woman is synonymous with being nurturing. Our culture ingrains us with the message: take care of others. Our caring nature and social expectations have led to exaggeration of this virtue. We have stretched our boundaries to become caretakers and rescuers. It is time to include ourselves in on the nurturing.

Keep Physically Active!

Most of my life I have been physically active because it's been fun. I enjoy it. I must admit, though, that in my mid-fifties, I find I need to exercise not only for the joy of it, but also for my health, to reduce stress and to balance my sedentary life as a therapist and author.

For too long women have looked at exercise with only calories in mind. Exercise does burn calories, but more importantly, exercise reduces the risk of osteoporosis, breast cancer, heart disease, and adult onset diabetes. It also relieves the symptoms of mild, chronic depression. Women need physical activity because it enhances self-esteem and reduces stress. You don't have to be overweight to need exercise.

Vigorous, continuous exercise consumes calories, and exercising for over 30 minutes means burning fat, but if improved health and well-being are your primary goals, exercising moderately and accumulatively will give you substantial health benefits, reduce your stress, and not impinge on your time. Review the tips in the chapter on exercise on how to fit moderate exercise into your routine.

Nutritional Health

As with exercise, monitor your dietary habits for good health and reduced stress, not just weight loss. Certainly, a sedentary life style implies eating less fat and fewer calories, but the focus is on good health and peace of mind, not self-deprivation.

Caffeine. If you are stressed, reduce your intake of caffeine (see Appendix A for the caffeine content of common foods and beverages) and sugar intake to prevent mood swings. Keep alert and mentally active by not overeating. Approximately half of all women who go to doctors go because they have some kind of pain in their breasts, usually caused by excess hormonal stimulation, excessive caffeine intake, or chronic stress (Northrup, 1994).

Fat. Reduce your risk of breast cancer, breast pain, and cyst formation by cutting fat intake to less than 20 percent. Reduce saturated fat to less than 10 percent and total fat to 20 percent if you have a family history of heart disease (Northrup, 1994).

Calcium. There are numerous reasons to take adequate amounts of calcium. Due to the exceedingly high risk of osteoporosis, especially as we age, calcium is a must for women. Because the amount of calcium in a woman's blood parallels the activities of the ovaries, there is a severe drop in blood calcium the week before menstruation and at the onset of menstruation. During menopause, the lack of ovarian hormones can cause severe calcium deficiency (Davis, 1970). The most prominent solution to osteoporosis (in addition to hormone replacement therapy and exercise) is increasing intake of calcium to the recommended dosages of at least 1,200 milligrams until you are 25, and approximately 800-1,000 mg thereafter—primarily from dairy products and calcium supplements.

However, getting an adequate amount of calcium involves more than just an increase in the amount of calcium you eat. Consider:

1. If your diet is too high in protein, the body draws calcium from the bones to counteract the acidity of your blood. The average American eats well in excess of the recommended 50 grams of protein daily (Northrup, 1994). Do you know your average daily intake of protein?

2. A diet high in fat contributes to decreased absorption of calcium (Northrup, 1994). Americans, on average, consume 40 percent of their calories as fat, well above the 20 to 30 percent recommended by a wide variety of nutrition experts and researchers.

Conclusion: If you are eating dairy products to increase your calcium intake, it is best to consume low-fat or nonfat dairy products. Since dairy products are also good sources of protein, you may need to monitor the amount of meat, poultry, or fish you consume because they also are high in protein. For good food sources of calcium see Appendix C. Consider:

1. Your body requires a ratio of 2:1 of calcium to magnesium.

2. Vitamin D increases the absorption of calcium. Increase absorption of calcium naturally by getting outside in the sun for twenty minutes daily, or drinking milk or other foods with added vitamin D.

Conclusion: Consider taking a calcium supplement that includes magnesium and vitamin D.

Sugar.   Reduce intake of sugar. It increases the excretion of calcium.

Fiber.   The National Cancer Institute recommends that we eat foods which provide 25 to 35 grams of fiber daily. At present Americans average 10 to 20 grams of fiber a day. Recent research indicates that foods high in fiber protect against colon cancer, diabetes, and coronary heart disease. Whole grains, legumes, fruits, and vegetables are high in fiber (Phillips, 1988).

Sodium.   Watch your sodium intake. For every 2,300 milligrams you consume, you excrete 40 to 80 milligrams of calcium. Reduce sodium to reduce risk of high blood pressure.

Food Pyramid = Optimal Health.   Gain optimal health (and loss of weight) by eating three moderate meals a day with additional healthy snacks mid-morning and mid-afternoon. The diet of choice advocated by most health professionals is a high fiber/high complex carbohydrate/low-fat diet. The emphasis is on complex carbohydrates—whole grains, pastas, breads, and legumes—comprising 70 percent of your diet. Eat plenty of fruits and vegetables—preferably fresh and whole. The following Pyramid Food Guide produced for the United States Department of Agriculture is an excellent source for helping you make healthy nutritional choices (Pawlak, 1993).

The allowances listed below are the Department of Agriculture's recommended daily allowances.

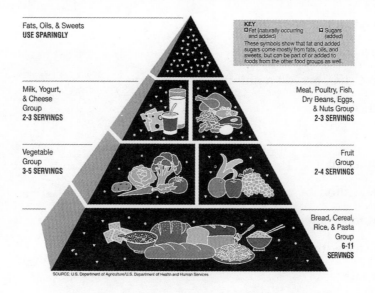

Food Group	Serving Size
Bread	1 slice bread, ½ bagel or English muffin, 1 oz. cold cereal, ½ oz. cooked cereal, rice or pasta, or 5-6 crackers.
Vegetable	1 cup raw, leafy vegetables, ½ cup cooked or chopped raw vegetables or ¾ cup vegetable juice.
Fruit	1 medium piece of fruit, ½ cup mixed fruit or ¾ cup of fruit juice.
Milk	1 cup milk or yogurt, 1 ½ oz. natural cheese or 2 oz. process cheese.
Meat	2-3 oz. cooked lean meat, poultry, or fish (the size of your fist). Other foods which count as 1 oz. of meat: ½ cup cooked dry beans, 1 egg, 2 tablespoons peanut butter, or ⅓ cup nuts.

Brush Up on Your Relaxation Skills

To be there for others, and to lend a helping hand and smile, is appropriate only if we can also say *no* without guilt. Our quality of giving improves when we allow time to meet our own needs. Unstructured personal time means alone time. It means your time to do what *you* want to do:

- Read
- Draw
- Listen to music
- Take a bubble bath
- Sit in a chair and do nothing
- Practice yoga
- T'ai chi
- Meditation
- Visualization
- Breathing exercises
- Have tea with a friend
- Fly a kite
- Do a cartwheel

It does not mean doing the laundry, or anything on your list of responsibilities. Some women use their personal time to catch up on the mounting pile of undone tasks. At times that is effective in reducing stress, but personal unstructured time is in addition to catching up on work.

Laughter is a wonderful antidote to stress. Joy is an art, don't leave it out of your life. Give yourself permission to play.

Women As Advocates and Role Models of Self-Care

Here are some examples of ways to incorporate self-care at work:

- Vote for candidates who enact legislation for walking trails and bike lanes.
- Support politicians who fight for improved standards of food inspection, honest labeling, and safety standards.
- Recommend fitness rooms and relaxation stations with ear phones for music or visualization at the job site.
- Advocate bonuses for non smokers and participants in exercise or Wellness Programs.
- Propose increasing availability of healthy snacks and beverages.
- Allocate a few minutes for relaxation skills, stretching, and eye exercises.

- Inspire others to use the stairs, bike to work, or get off the bus one stop early by example!

- Exhort a friend to pair up for a walk during part of the lunch break.

- Bring in a low-fat protein snack for a mid-afternoon pick-me-up.

You are your children's primary role model. Encourage an active life style for your children. According to the President's Council on Fitness, American children are getting slower, weaker, and fatter, while watching too much television, eating too much fast food, and getting too little exercise (1993b). Encourage active weekends as a family: when going to the park for picnics, include pitching a baseball or hiking around the lake. Go with the kids on a bike ride, or swim with them. If you only watch them play, you miss out on the exercise and fun, and become a role model of inactivity.

Let your full potential flower. Be yourself, take time for yourself, enjoy yourself, express yourself, take care of yourself.

—— INCORPORATING SELF-CARE AT WORK AND HOME ——

Look over the lists of ideas above for both personal unstructured time and advocating self-care at work. Use them or create your own list of ways you plan to incorporate more self-care into your life.

Personal Time

1. _____
2. _____
3. _____

At Work

1. _____
2. _____
3. _____

The following chapter will help you create your own personalized Wellness Program. Incorporate these self-care plans and other techniques you have learned in this chapter into your Wellness Program.

22

Creating Your Own
Wellness Program

*The aspiration to improve ourselves, to reach out constantly
toward a greater goal, is available to all of us if we are willing to
recapture those strengths that are part of our natural
heritage—our potential to be well, our potential for choice,
self-healing, self-direction, and self-mastery.*

—Patricia Norris quoted in
Healers on Healing

You are ready to create a Wellness Program that will work for you whenever you feel stressed, anxious, or depressed. In Part I you determined what triggers your stress at work and how you respond to it physically, emotionally, and behaviorally. In Part II you learned a wide range of stress management techniques. You also learned how to transform defeatism into positive self-esteem, to see obstacles as challenges, and to change negative moods by correcting distorted thinking. Now you have the opportunity to combine your Stress Profile from Part I with the stress management techniques from Part II that you've found to be most effective and enjoyable into a comprehensive Wellness Program.

Your Stress Resiliency

Your Wellness Program will both reduce your current stress and build your stress resiliency. Wellness in body, mind, and spirit will give you a resilience to all the stresses you face in your day-to-day life. Active stress prevention as a life style strengthens your immune system and boosts your spirits, enabling you to meet the trials of life successfully. Eating well, exercising, appreciating yourself, getting enough sleep, providing personal time, relaxing, and adopting the other healthy stress management techniques taught in Part II result in a Hardiness Personality. You have the tools to live life with enthusiasm, commitment, and self-assurance.

Reviewing Your Stress Management Skills

The following list reviews all of the stress management techniques you learned in Part II. As you go over the list, check those you plan to use or are currently using. Space is provided for you to be specific: such as particular office stretches you are using, or concrete dietary changes you have made or plan to make. If needed, refer to the summary exercises you completed at the end of each chapter in Part II.

1. Relaxation Skills

    _____ a. Conscious Breathing

    _____ b. Deep Relaxation (Active and Passive)

    _____ c. Visualization

    Your favorite application(s): _____

    _____

2. Meditation

    _____ a. Meditating (using one word/phrase)

    _____ b. Quiet Time/Recreation

    _____ c. Creative Time

    _____ d. Journaling

    Your favorite application(s): _____

    _____

3. Exercise

    _____ a. Physical activity (aerobic or accumulated)

_____ b. Office stretching routines (full or mini-routines)

Your favorite application(s): _____

_____

4. Nutrition

_____ a. Alternative Foods (to stress/food snacking)

_____ b. Alternative activities

_____ c. Stress management diet tips

Your favorite application(s): _____

_____

5. Reframing Your Thinking

_____ a. Four Steps to Change Negative Thinking

_____ b. Worry Break/Worry Focus

Your favorite application(s): _____

_____

6. Feelings and Communication Skills

_____ a. Three Steps to Reduce Anxiety, Depression, Anger

_____ b. Assertive Communication Styles (I-Statements, Scripting)

_____ c. Good Listening Styles (Attentive, Disarming, Supporting)

Your favorite application(s): _____

_____

7. Social Support

_____ a. Increasing support at work (with coworkers, management)

_____ b. Increasing support outside work (with family, friends, groups)

Your favorite application(s): _____

_____

8. Self-Care (especially for working women)

_____ a. Self-Nurturing (giving yourself a "gift")

_____ b. Personal time (time to do anything you want or nothing at all!)

Your favorite application(s): _____

_____

—————— YOUR WELLNESS PROGRAM ——————

Using your Stress Profile from Part I, select your most troublesome job stressors and predominant stress symptoms to fill in the blanks below. Next, using the list of selected stress management techniques you just compiled, choose the most relevant and effective responses to your work stressors and symptoms.

Below is an example from my files to guide you. Vickie came to me feeling overwhelmed by job stress and on the verge of giving up hope of coping with her work situation. After practicing all of the stress management techniques, she created her own Wellness Program. After several weeks of consistent practice, she was surprised and pleased with how much better she felt.

Vickie's Wellness Program

Vickie's Work Situation

Vickie had just been promoted—the first female employee in her company to become personnel manager of Development and Research. The problem was that the person she was now reporting to was someone she had been avoiding.

Vickie's Work Stressor(s)

1. Inharmonious work relationship

2. Promotion

Vickie's Stress Symptoms

Physical: Sleepless after 3 a.m.; flare-up of an old back injury

Emotional: Highly anxious and tense

Behavioral: Snapping at her kids, inattentive to husband. Creativity and concentration at work diminished. No new ideas in weeks.

Vickie's Selected Stress Management Techniques

1. Changing Negative Self-Talk

Using the Four Steps to Changing Negative Thinking Vickie wrote down her self-talk regarding her inharmonious work relationship. "I am unable to do the job because of the tension between me and my boss. How can I? He is already condescending to me and was rude to me numerous times even before my promotion." Vickie found her self-talk contained thinking distortions she could change. She adjusted her self-talk to a more neutral view. She then worked on accepting that she could not change the situation and instead focused on ways she could reduce her own anxiety and stress.

2. Relaxation Skills

Vickie began using Conscious Breathing and Deep Relaxation with Visualization to calm her nerves at work. Several times during her work day she would take three Complete Breaths and visualize sitting beside a waterfall. As a reminder to take these breaks, she hung a picture of a waterfall in her new office.

3. Exercise

Vickie created a mini-routine for her back from the office stretching routines and practiced it once an hour. She reinstated her back exercises at home.

4. Journaling

Vickie bought a notebook, and on the train ride home from work, she did some writing to explore her emotions toward her boss and his behavior.

5. Feelings and Communication Skills

Vickie learned more about herself and her contribution to the tension by applying the circle exercise from Reducing Your Anger at Work. She then focused on assertiveness skills that would keep her conversation with her boss on task. She developed a listening style to disarm and deflect any unjust criticism from him.

Results:

Vickie and her boss established a satisfactory working relationship. Her anxiety symptoms diminished, her back pain subsided, and her creativity and enthusiasm for her work returned.

Now it is your turn to apply your selected stress management techniques to your specific work stressors to create your own Wellness Program. Begin by selecting what you want to focus on from your Stress Profile.

Your Work Situation: _____

_____

_____

_____

_____

Your Work Stressor(s):

1. _____

2. _____

3. _____

Your Stress Symptoms:

Physical: _____

_____

_____

Emotional: _____

_____

_____

Behavioral: _____

_____

_____

Your Selected Stress Management Techniques

Use the space below to select and describe the skills you plan to apply from any or all of the eight categories (relaxation skills; meditation; exercise; nutrition; reframing your thinking; feelings and communication; social support; and self-care).

1. _____

_____

_____

2. _____

_____

_____

3. _____

_____

_____

4. _____

_____

_____

5. _____

_____

6. _____

_____

_____

7. _____

_____

_____

8. _____

_____

_____

After applying your Wellness Program at work for several weeks, return to this space and record how your stress symptoms have been reduced and other examples of your success. Enjoy your good feelings and congratulate yourself!

Results:

Conclusion

The goal of your Wellness Program is to build resiliency to stress. We find better solutions when we *change* ourselves and *take care* of ourselves. We then tackle problems from a place of inner strength and harmony. By developing our resources and reserves, the outer stress is diminished relative to our inner growth, allowing us to handle greater stress levels. The final step to wellness at work is the personal resolve to maintain these new skills and habits of health and well-being.

23

Personal Commitment—The Key

It is effort that brings us to greatness and the fusion of what we are with what we can be.

—Dr. George Sheehan quoted in *Adventure
Athletes: Runners and Walkers*

The *Wellness at Work* stress management and behavioral techniques are seminal sources of wellness—but the key to wellness is your own firm resolve to do what it takes! The tools for optimal health and happiness are now yours. The quality of your life depends on regular practice of these self-help tools. This is the most difficult aspect of wellness—forging the discipline needed to practice habits of well-being.

Each of us needs to flip the inner switch of will, to take charge and do what is essential. No one else can tell us when or how to change. It is an internal decision for happiness. If you use your inner strength to overturn old habits, you will find victory and joy. You will feel satisfied and full of enthusiasm when you live the essentials of a healthy life style. The wellness approach to life both prevents and cures stress. Your Wellness Program will enable you to move from living at the turbulent edge of yourself to expressing yourself at work and in every aspect of your life from the peaceful, strong center within you.

How do you activate the process? When willpower is expressed as determination, there is implied a grit that dominates for a period of time—a battle of internal forces. Often determination gradually succumbs to the strength of old habits. The real strength of the will is self-motivation. When your "shoulds" and "ought to" statements about wellness become "I want," "I choose," and "I am" statements, you have unlocked a powerful force which emanates from a willingness and enthusiasm—*choice* encompassing full intent. Then the will is a flowing process, a natural strength.

Good health and inner harmony are products of healthy living habits. We are constantly making choices that result in peace of mind and vibrant health—or ill health and mental anguish.

Ask yourself:

- Am I willing to make a commitment to wellness and self-care?

- Am I ready to discipline myself to exercise, eat nutritiously, and practice relaxation techniques consistently?

- Will the overwhelmingly supportive data, substantial financial savings, and promise of improved personal well-being and health be sufficient to motivate me to stick to preventative health care?

Over 53 percent of the deaths in this country are caused by life style decisions which are self-destructive and negligent behaviors, such as smoking, drinking, driving without seat belts, driving under the influence of alcohol or drugs, noncompliance with physicians' prescriptions, eating fatty foods, and not exercising (Witmer and Sweeney, 1992). The "quick fix" success of medication or surgery allows the patient to return to old habits without apparent penalty. A "fix me" attitude lets the patient get away with a passive role in his health care, but only for a while. For example, continuing to smoke after lung cancer surgery is not good for longevity!

Gradually Americans are awakening to the shortcomings of such an approach. More and more people are willing to commit to life style changes and to take charge of their personal wellness. Over 50 million Americans have turned to alternative (also called complementary) therapy for relief. According to a New England Journal of Medicine report, "U.S. patients made 425 million visits to alternative caregivers in 1990 compared with 388 million visits to family doctors and internists" (Eisenberg et al., 1993). Nutrition, exercise, biofeedback, meditation, homeopathy, and relaxation techniques now complement more conventional treatments such as psychotherapy, psychotropic medication, vaccines, and surgery. The alternative therapies are highly beneficial in the reduction of stress whether on or off the job. This new integrated approach to health blends the best of traditional science with preventative and wellness oriented therapies.

The federal approach to health care is historically corrective rather than preventative. The federal government spends 75 percent of its health care dollars caring for people with chronic illnesses and less than one percent on prevention of occurrence of these same diseases (Witmer and Sweeney, 1992). There is a change developing. In 1992 the National Institute of Health established an Office of Alternative Medicine, which may presage a positive expansion of federal health care philosophy. The goal of the Office is to evaluate alternative or unconventional medical treatments, and to provide information to the public about them (Office of Alternative Medicine, 1992). In addition, the United Nations 1993 World Labor Report directly supports alternative approaches to counteract stress, including breathing exercises, meditation and mental imagery, progressive muscle relaxation, exercise, and nutrition (International Labor Office, 1993).

Corporate encouragement can help to a great extent. For example, on-site Wellness Programs, corporate bonuses to non smokers, short stretching or relaxation breaks, and availability of nutritious snacks all help to reduce mental barriers or resistance to self-care. More information on the ways management can contribute to wellness at work is located in Part IV.

There is only one real solution to this largely self-created epidemic of ill health: preventative action. Healthy living is the number one weapon against physical illness, mental anxiety, and depression. Self-care, including good nutrition, exercise, and enjoyable relaxation, is commonsense stress management.

Testimonials by people who have used the simple but powerful techniques of *Wellness at Work* abound. Their lives have been changed. "Why did I wait so long?" they exclaim, and, "I had to experience it to believe it!" Their smiling eyes and quiet surety express their success.

Part III

Professional Services

24

Knowing Your Mental
Health Benefits

*The more accepting you become of yourself, the more you can see
others in the same light.*

—Joan Borysenko, *Minding the Body,
Mending the Mind*

An Employee Assistance Program (EAP) is a mental health service program offered to employees by their employer. EAP benefits are in addition to your major medical coverage, and typically are for office visits for outpatient mental health counseling.

EAPs were initially established as an answer to occupational alcoholism in the 1940s. If a supervisor found that alcoholism interfered with job performance, he would refer the employee to the EAP. As employers have come to recognize the impact of unresolved personal issues on job performance, EAP services have expanded to include issues ranging from drug and alcohol abuse, to marital and family issues, job stress, anger management, depression, and anxiety. Although an employer can and does refer employees for counseling due to impaired job performance, more and more people seek counseling through their EAP on a self-referred basis (U.S. Department of Health and Human Services, 1990).

Although EAP mental health benefits for employees are inadequate, and at times a stop gap measure at best, there is a growing interest, concern, and commitment by employers and management to develop or expand EAPs to meet the needs of employees. EAP psychotherapists are also encouraging employees to utilize psychotherapy in conjunction with Wellness Programs, group counseling, and self-help approaches such as those detailed in Part II. Therapy also works well when coupled with free local support groups such as Alcoholics Anonymous (AA), Overeaters Anonymous (OA), and Women's Domestic Violence Coalition. Primary care physicians are increasingly referring to and working with mental health practitioners.

Reasons Why Employees Under-Utilize EAPs

There are five important reasons why employees fail to make full use of mental health benefits available to them.

1. *Employees' Lack of Knowledge of EAP Benefits.* Although four out of five illnesses are stress-related, and up to 80 percent of a primary care physician's practice is made up of patients with stress-related illnesses, employees are often uninformed regarding their mental health benefits.

Overcome your lack of knowledge about EAPs; find out the specific benefits of your company's EAP. Speak with your EAP representative, or review available literature. Whether or not your company has an EAP, you may have psychiatric coverage and outpatient mental health (counseling) coverage under your health insurance. Investigate your major medical insurance. The following is an example of how to utilize both EAP and major medical insurance.

> *John, an employee of Appleton Furniture Inc., was experiencing depression due to a family crisis and it was affecting his productivity at work. He was referred to his company's EAP to see a Marriage Family Child Counselor for the allotted five free sessions. Both he and his therapist recognized his need for further counseling. If he had been in crisis and needed psychiatric care or hospitalization, he would have checked his benefits under his major medical insurance. Since John was not in crisis but needed continued psychotherapy, he needed to find out whether an outpatient mental health coverage was within his major medical health insurance plan.*

Most major medical insurance plans include mental health provisions. They vary from crisis intervention only, to weekly, long-term psychotherapy.

If your company does not have an EAP, discuss Chapter 25 with your manager or employer; it portrays the financial benefits of EAPs and Wellness Programs for employers. Mental health services for employees benefit employers as well.

2. *Fear of Psychotherapy.* It takes courage to go to a psychotherapist for the first time. It is especially difficult if you do not know what to expect. The therapist begins by actively listening and validating what you are experiencing. At the beginning of his first session one

client stated, "I don't need your advice." But he did need me to listen. Initially, stressed clients need a safe, neutral yet supportive setting to air their distress. As noted psychologist Carl Rogers put it, the patient needs, and hopefully receives from any therapist, "unconditional positive regard."

At times there may be a mismatch in personalities or style of therapy. If you are not satisfied with the therapeutic approach being taken to your problem or there is a personality mismatch, try another therapist.

The following is a general description of a first session of therapy. Much of this session is standard within the profession, although personalities and modalities do lead to some differences. The therapist's job is to find out why you are there, whether it is the stressful situation, the symptoms of stress, or both. The initial part of therapy focuses on the following questions.

- Why are you seeking counseling at this particular time? What made you call now, today?

- Was there a precipitating event or increase in intensity of stress? For example, were you just notified of an unwanted transfer, did your spouse leave you, or was a major car repair the last straw?

- If there was not a specific stressor or event that triggered your need for help, perhaps it was a growing awareness of symptoms of stress such as an inability to sleep, recurrent nightmares, or inability to concentrate.

- Have you seen a therapist before?

- Have you had or are you currently on psychotropic medication? Is there relevant medical history?

- What is your history or current usage of drugs and/or alcohol?

- The therapist may ask for a very brief overview of your current family situation, and in this or the next session, a brief description of your family of origin and early life experiences.

- The therapist usually asks, "What are your goals for therapy? What do you hope to gain from therapy?" You and the therapist formulate a treatment plan.

Often a person who comes into counseling is highly stressed and requires immediate help. The therapist needs to assess the severity of the problem and initiate therapeutic assistance. Hands-on practical advice is given to alleviate the client's present pain. In addition to being a good listener, the therapist helps the client learn how to cope with the current stressful situation. The advice could range from recommending you see your primary care physician (or a psychiatrist if medication is indicated), to teaching you a relaxation technique or encouraging you to reestablish an exercise routine. The therapist begins the process of helping you regain your own self-worth.

One of my clients who is also active in AA, told me, "Therapy is an oasis, a safe haven where I can gain insight about myself and my relationships." Counseling offers the opportunity for you to regroup and gain skills for living a fuller, more enriching life.

3. *Fear of Social Stigma or Financial Penalties.* You may be avoiding therapy because you are worried that fellow workers may learn of your being in therapy. Confidentiality is not only a strict standard of the profession, but mandated by law. Therapists may not divulge the names of their clients or the content of sessions without the client's permission. Therapists are required to get a signed release by the client before consulting with psychiatrists, primary care physicians, school counselors, or others. Legal exceptions to this rule exist where there is an imminent danger of suicide or homicide, child abuse, or a court subpoena of records.

To be certain of the confidentiality rule in your area, get clarification on your state's legal position from a therapist, state mental health official, or other authority. Also get clarification at work. Obviously there may be stricter confidentiality standards in private practice or in EAPs run by a Health Maintenance Organization (HMO) that administers the company's major medical and mental health services, than an EAP administered in-house. The intent of confidentiality is the same, but with progress reports and other paper work, required doctor's referrals, or counseling resulting from a referral by a supervisor or manager, it is harder to maintain strict confidentiality. At times, the *fact* that you are in counseling is known, but not the content of the sessions.

4. *Avoidance.* Under-utilization can be due to an employee's avoidance of the signals of need for help. Busy schedules, growing responsibilities, and financial and time constraints often cause people to ignore such signals as inability to sleep, indigestion, anxiety, depression, interpersonal tensions, and a host of other emotional and physical warning signs. Counseling seems like "too much of a bother." People mutter, "I can tough it out" or "It will go away." Avoiding counseling also serves to obscure the fact that "the other guy" is only half the problem.

5. *Limitations of EAPs.* Some employees refuse EAP services because the coverage is brief. Many allow only three to five sessions per year, per family member. Do not be fooled by time constraints. Even a few sessions can break a negative pattern and get you back on track. The traditional approach of long-term therapy is being replaced with brief therapy. Many therapists are educating their clients in new ways of viewing themselves and the world, and teaching practical behavioral skills to improve self-care, relaxation, communication, and self-esteem. Recent research indicates that 75 percent of the time the presenting problem of the client can be resolved in eight sessions. If a couple with one child saw an EAP therapist for their allotted three sessions each, there would be more than a 75 percent chance of success!

Sessions can be combined to meet the unique situation of each family. For example, with one client family of four, where the EAP granted each family member three sessions, I saw the parent as a couple for two sessions and individually for two sessions; then the whole family for four sessions; their two teenage boys individually and together for three sessions; and finished with a final family session. Total: twelve sessions. In the case of that family, improved communication and parenting skills coupled with clearing up old hurts greatly improved family dynamics.

If issues are more complex, a program which offers longer coverage and low co-payments can provide more time for changes to take root. For example, I was counseling a family through a marital separation complicated by their teenage son's Defiant Conduct Disorder. EAP benefits of five sessions per family and co-payments of $40 brought the counseling to a halt. A month later the family returned because the corporation changed to an EAP which provided broader coverage for their employees. The added time with them, provided by reduced co-payments and an increased allotment of sessions, allowed them to work through complex issues and achieve a family reconciliation.

Types of Mental Health Care Providers

There are specific, highly technical definitions and requirements (which vary from state to state) for the following types of mental health care providers. The following are general descriptions.

A. Psychotherapist

The terms psychotherapist and psychotherapy are generic terms covering mental health counselors and counseling in general and can be applied to any of the following mental health care providers. At times the terms are shortened to therapist and therapy.

B. Psychiatrist

Psychiatrists have training similar to MDs, the area of specialization being mental pathology. By license and training they can administer medication, and are the only mental health care providers so licensed. Some psychiatrists have a full counseling practice, while most focus on diagnosis and medication management, leaving the counseling to the other mental health care providers. Psychiatry is covered under your major medical benefits.

C. Psychologist

Psychologists have a doctoral degree (Ph.D.) in psychology. In addition to counseling skills, they are trained in psychological testing.

D. Marriage Family Child Counselor (MFCC)

MFCCs counsel individuals, couples, families, or groups. With additional training, MFCCs may elect to administer psychological testing. MFCCs train people in anger management, parenting skills, and communication skills. They offer techniques in stress reduction and ways to increase self-esteem and curb addictions.

E. Licensed Clinical Social Worker (LCSW)

LCSWs are trained as social workers and then can elect to be licensed for counseling. They are on a par with MFCCs. There is little difference in their approach to counseling from MFCCs.

F. Fitness and Wellness Programs

Fitness and Wellness Programs are wonderful ways to increase your understanding of stress. They offer an excellent means for learning and experiencing coping skills. Whether it is an on-site aerobics class or a lecture on stress management, communication skills, or nutrition, these programs are useful methods for defusing accumulated stress. They can be an adjunct to your own Wellness Program or an inspiration for change. They also provide a means of socializing with coworkers in a relaxed and informal manner. See Chapter 25 for statistics on how these programs improve your health and well-being.

Conclusion

Mental health services, including EAPs, Wellness Programs, private therapy, and support groups are wonderful resources. We all have periods in our lives when we are highly stressed. Just as it is beneficial to have a primary care physician and dentist, it is helpful to know what is available to you for mental health. Review your mental health benefits under your insurance plan if you have one, find out more about your EAP, and discover what services are available to you in your area. In this way, if there is a need, you and your family will know where to turn for help.

Professional services provide an avenue for you to gain a clearer perspective of yourself. They are a means for you to learn how better to handle the stresses you may be confronting. Their primary purpose is to help you become more aware of your own inner strengths.

Part IV

For Managers and Employers

25

EAPs and Wellness Programs:
Sound Investments

*The companies which are likely to be the most successful in the
future are those which help employees cope with stress and also
carefully re-engineer the workplace to make it better suited to
human aptitudes and aspirations.*

—1993 U.N. World Labor Report

So far, every word in this book applies to anyone who works for a company, regardless of
the shade of one's collar or whether the uniform is a three piece suit or coveralls. This section
is especially for the owners and managers who have a special responsibility to bring wellness
to the workplace.

Wellness at work means satisfied workers *and* high productivity. Wellness at work
means healthy working relationships *and* healthy profits. The financial well-being of a
company goes hand-in-hand with employee well-being. This is truer today than ever before,
and any manager who ignores this axiom does so at the company's risk.

The cost of employee stress is astronomical and growing rapidly—and today its
reduction is one of the most financially attractive investments any business can make.
Consider the following.

- In California alone, stress-related claims for workers' compensation increased 700 percent between 1979 and 1988. Nine out of ten claims resulted in payment. In 1989, $380 million was paid to California workers for such stress-related problems as sleeplessness and headaches (California Workers' Compensation Institute, 1990). Due to a January 1994 ruling tightening the criteria and burden of proof, workers' stress claims in California are becoming less plentiful and less successful.

- American industry loses approximately $19.4 billion in production time because of premature coronary death and pays $15 billion for employee sick leave. General Motors spends more for employee health care than it does for the purchase of steel (Cooper, 1978)!

- American employers are spending an estimated $700 billion a year to replace people who have quit work before retirement age because of stress-related coronary heart disease (International Labor Office, 1993).

- Troubled employees who are not in recovery or counseling programs are costly— the employer pays approximately 25 percent of an alcoholic's annual salary due to dollars lost through absenteeism, lowered productivity, and increased medical coverage (Jones, 1980).

- A major cause of absenteeism is depression, costing employers an estimated $17 billion in 1989 (Castro, 1993).

- One in four American adults are troubled by anxiety or depression, with half of these people facing the added stress of alcohol or drug abuse (Regier et al., 1993).

For the sake of the businesses, not to mention other reasons, these people need help. Medical experts and business executives agree that increased mental health coverage would pay for itself. For example, the National Institute of Mental Health estimates that lithium alone has saved the U.S. economy $40 billion since 1970 by making it possible for those who are severely depressed to stabilize and return to work (Castro, 1993). Therapy and antidepressants help people through such painful situations as separation and divorce which could result in lost days at work, a financial stress to both the employer and employee.

What can you as an employer do to ease the pain of stress for the employee and at the same time increase productivity? Is it time for you to implement an EAP or Wellness Program? Below are statistics on the financial benefits of EAPs for the employer, and guidelines for establishing an EAP or Wellness Program.

Cost-Benefit Ratios Favor EAPs

EAPs are cost-effective. For example, the Kimberly-Clark Corporation showed a 70 percent decrease in on-the-job accidents with their program. General Motors reported a 40 percent reduction in lost time and a 60 percent decrease in sickness and accident benefits. The Equitable Life Insurance Society and the Kennecot Corporation estimate that they have achieved a return of approximately six dollars for each dollar invested in their Employee Assistance Programs (International Labor Office, 1993).

One study, an independently conducted cost-benefit analysis of McDonnell Douglas Corporation's EAP, establishes that a well-managed EAP is singularly the most effective way to manage health care costs related to psychiatric care and substance abuse. In the analysis of costs associated with health care claims and absenteeism for a multi-year period before and after EAP intervention, the EAP annual cost savings minus annual program operating expenses was $2.5 million in 1987 and 3.9 million in 1988. This represents nearly a 3:1 return on investment in 1987 and over a 4:1 return on investment in 1988. This study used accepted statistical and scientific methods, analyzed a large number of employees (approximately 5,000), and covered a three year period. This conservative study used only two cost variables: actual health claims costs and absenteeism, both of which can be accurately measured. Less easily measurable factors such as productivity, job-performance level, and other subjective data were not analyzed (*The Almacan*, 1989).

EAPs can substantially increase profits as well as improve employee health and well-being. More and more employers are establishing EAPs for their employees. Corporate America is increasingly recognizing that personal problems affect employee job performance. A nationwide survey of 508 human-resource professionals and 502 working adults shows 92 percent of employees and 93 percent of management agree that personal problems contribute to difficulties at work. It has been estimated that approximately 80 percent of the Fortune 500 companies have incorporated an EAP or behavioral health program in the last five to seven years (King, 1995).

Smaller companies may lack the resources to establish an in-house EAP. Most EAP experts agree that 200 employees is the minimum number of employees required for an in-house effort. Often companies pool their resources to create health packages which give greater benefits at reduced co-payments (cost to the employee). One solution is for smaller companies to band together and develop a consortium, subcontracting services from an existing program or contracting with a Health Maintenance Organization or Preferred Provider Organization (U.S. Department of Health and Human Services, 1990).

Wellness Programs

Employee fitness programs are another excellent means of facilitating good health, reducing stress, improving job performance and productivity, and reducing soaring health care costs.

The first true employee fitness program was established at the National Cash Register Company in Dayton, Ohio, in 1894. The program consisted of morning and afternoon exercise breaks for employees. Over the years, other major corporations followed suit. Today, successful employee programs abound, including ones at Apple Computer, Dow Chemical,

Proctor and Gamble, Pacific Bell, Pepsico, Chase Manhattan Bank, Xerox, Travelers Insurance Company, and Tenneco, to mention a few. At Tenneco, the average annual medical claim for a non-exercising female employee ($1,535) was more than twice that of women who participated in the in-house exercise program ($639). For men, the average claim for non-exercisers ($1,003) was nearly twice that of exercisers ($561) (President's Council, 1993c).

According to Dr. Herbert Benson, MD, associate professor of medicine at Harvard Medical School and president of the Mind/Body Institute of New England Deaconess Hospital, "Instituting a stress management program can reduce physician's office visits by as much as 50 percent . . . [B]y shifting health care to self-care, people will not only feel better and more empowered, but it will also save money" (Walker, 1991).

Dr. Kenneth Cooper, MD, has gathered extensive data clearly demonstrating that effective Wellness Programs reduce health care premiums, increase productivity, decrease absenteeism, reduce turnover, and improve worker morale. Dr. Cooper is a recognized authority on Wellness Programs and author of numerous books on the benefits of exercise, nutrition, and stress management. At the Cooper Aerobics Institute in Dallas he encourages a healthy life style through his Life-Links Wellness Program which awards up to $400 in annual bonuses for employees who work out at the clinic's health club and attend lectures on nutrition and stress reduction (Cooper, 1978).

The Importance of Management Support

The attitude of management towards fitness can have a major impact on employees. Encouragement and support from the top for a healthy life style can be contagious. A strong leadership role, including personal participation in exercise, sound nutrition, and stress management practices, results in enthusiastic involvement by employees.

Costs for employee fitness programs vary greatly. It may be as little as the cost of a "paper program" with bulletins, newsletters, and other fitness literature, or as much as millions of dollars for an extensive in-house facility. Even a paper program can be effective. No matter what the size of the company, leadership can encourage physical activity by employees.

Over 40 percent of corporations with 50 or more employees have introduced on-site exercise programs (President's Council, 1993c). One such company, Canada Life Assurance Company and North American Life Assurance Company, found that regular physical fitness programs for managers resulted in a 3 percent rise in productivity and a 22 percent reduction in absenteeism. In the United States, Control Data found that health care costs halved for those in a cardiovascular fitness program as compared to those not in the program (International Labor Office, 1993).

Healthy, stress-free employees are a vital investment in the future success of your company. Managers are well advised to take an active role in employee physical and mental well-being.

26

For Management: Four Keys to Easing Employee Stress

Few things help an individual more than to place responsibility upon him, and to let him know you trust him.

—Booker T. Washington

Catch people in the act of doing something right.

—Ken Blanchard, *The One-Minute Manager*

There are four keys to dynamic wellness held by managers and owners of businesses both large and small. They are keys to increased employee job satisfaction, higher productivity, decreased absenteeism, and lower health costs. None of them are very expensive to implement, and all of them can give your business benefits far out of proportion to their cost. They should be thought of as major business opportunities. They are as follows:

1. *Maximize flexibility* in your organization so that employees can synchronize their lives with company needs rather than feel boxed in.

2. *Keep employees well-informed* as to company policy, procedure, and goals to reduce doubts and worries.

3. *Make employees part of the decision-making process* so that they don't feel controlled by a system that gives orders from the top down.

4. *Enhance employee self-esteem* through well-considered company policies and practices.

Here are the keys in greater detail.

Four Keys to Employee Wellness

Maximize Flexibility

Rigid work schedules can have a significant impact on the psychological and physical health of your employees. In my counseling practice I repeatedly hear clients designate rigid scheduling as their primary stressor at work. Arbitrary assignment of vacation schedules, unpredictable rotating shifts, and permanent night shifts result in emotional distress.

> *Joe walked into my office and sat down. Ringing his hands and with eyes riveted to the floor, he exclaimed, "I'm boxed in. I have no choices. Where is the flexibility? Where is the consideration for individual needs and preferences? I feel trapped. Cindy and I are both working full time, but with one kid in day care and the other in kindergarten, we need some flexibility in our work schedules. Where is the heart? Where is the caring?"*

My heart reached out to him and his plight. Joe and Cindy are part of a new generation of workers who require a variety of choices. Dual-working parents, the single working parent, working students, and older workers need alternatives to the five-day week, eight-hour day, nine-to-five schedule. Employers need to recognize employee demands and responsibilities outside the work site, and introduce flexibility into the workplace. To reduce stress and improve morale, employers must be sensitive to employee concerns, including family and parenting issues.

Over 20 million families in the United States have children aged thirteen years or younger. Nearly two-thirds of all families have at least two wage earners, and 54 percent of all women are in the work force (U.S. Department of Labor, 1993). These statistics highlight a special need for improvements in the workplace regarding child care. The tension of leaving children in inadequate or inconsistent situations results in low productivity, low morale, and absenteeism.

Flexible starting and quitting times (within limits set by management) and compressed work weeks where employees can work four ten-hour days rather than five eight-hour days are two positive management responses. Other creative responses by companies have been to institute part-time employment that includes prorated benefits, job security, and all other rights available to the company's full-time workers, or job sharing, where two people share one full-time position, with benefits and salary prorated.

An alternative to layoffs is to institute work sharing, in which all or part of an organization's work force temporarily reduces hours and salary (New Ways to Work Publications, 1993). Other opportunities for flexibility may occur depending on the nature of the job. If you are a supervisor, a manager, or an owner of a company, ask: what can I do to increase flexibility for the employee and at the same time increase productivity?

Open Communication

Nancy came into my office during her lunch break. "I am so mixed up," she confessed. "God, I am thrilled on one level. This is the third in a series of major layoffs and I haven't been cut. In my department of ten, there are only five of us left. But what about Jean and the others? Some of them have more financial pressures than I do. What are they going to do? Joe's wife has cancer, and Molly and her husband just took on a large mortgage. I feel so guilty. What did I do to survive? Why am I one of the lucky ones? I can't even sleep with all this uncertainty. I wish they'd tell me what's happening."

Downsizing, layoffs, and economic insecurity are all part of economic reality. In a climate of intense competition, employee job security is tenuous, job obsolescence is a threat, and forced retirement is commonplace.

For example, in 1985 General Motors began reducing its work force from 132,000 employees to a 1993 level of 71,000 employees, a drop of 47 percent. Annual costs have been cut 1.5 billion in the last year. According to Tony Hain, Ph.D., psychologist and director of human resources for General Motors, from 1991 to 1992, 1.5 million employees in Canada and the United States lost their jobs due to downsizing (Adler, 1993a). Salaried employees are losing their jobs at a rate of 2,500 per working day. In the past, downsizing primarily affected blue-collar workers. Now white-collar workers, especially middle management, are affected. Only 10 percent are able to find a job as good as they had before, and most new jobs are part-time or temporary (Adler, 1993b). Downsizing may be necessary for economic survival, but the stress is compounded if it is handled in a tight-lipped and arbitrary manner. Nothing is more stressful than having this difficult process carried out in a secretive and unthinking or unfair manner (real or imagined). There is tremendous stress on employees due to lack of information. Rumor-infested gossip makes problems worse. Employee insecurity causes fear, loss of motivation and commitment, depression, and anxiety, even when an employee continues on the job.

These stressors understandably cause anxiety, insomnia, depression, and other stress symptoms. Laying off people to cut costs is successful only if it can be accomplished with a minimum of stress for those who survive the cuts. It is the responsibility of management to minimize the stress inherent in times of economic insecurity.

The most humane and tension-reducing approach is for management to keep employees well informed. Open lines of communication are imperative, including meetings for employees to vent fears and have questions answered. The agonizing tension inherent in the situation can be minimized by keeping the employees well informed of each step of the process: why, when, and how the company is downsizing. It is vital for the health of the downsizing company to do so in a sensitive, fair, and open manner.

Some of the successful strategies which ease the stress of downsizing include: opening lines of communication, not hiring new employees, offering early retirement or lucrative incentives to leave, redesigning positions, job sharing, and partial retirement.

IBM's approach serves as an excellent example of successful downsizing. In 1986 it had 407,000 employees worldwide, and by the end of 1993, only 277,000 employees. Although survivors of the layoffs were deeply stressed, the situation was eased by IBM's clarification of its need to downsize and provision of constantly updated information for the employees. Downsizing pressures were ameliorated through lucrative retirements, buy-out packages, relocation of willing workers, choice of lower positions, and communication (Adler, 1993b). Can these ideas be applied creatively in your firm?

Employee Participation in Decision-Making

The most significant move a business can make to reduce stress, particularly anxiety and depression, is to allow employees a voice in the decision-making process. One of the most common features of both anxiety and depression is a sense of no longer being in control of one's life.

> **Hank** started talking even before he took a seat. "I am bummed. Here I am in middle management, but do I have a say? No! My supervisor keeps telling me what to do and how to run my team. She commanded me to write up a formal complaint on one of my team members. She won't even listen to what I have to say. I don't agree with her, and it's my neck on the line, and my signature on the document. What am I supposed to do? I'm caught in the middle. You know, I'm not working for the money alone and neither is my team. I believe in trust and respect. My supervisor thinks everyone is out to cut corners and do as little as necessary. But no, my team agrees with me. Driving us, pressuring us, not trusting or respecting us, and not including us in the decision-making process decrease our productivity and enthusiasm for our job. What can I do?"
>
> Hank decided to look at all his options and their consequences before choosing his response. He chose to file the report with additional documentation of his position. He also worked to improve his ability to voice his opinion without getting angry or blaming others.

Typically, the person feels that options have been narrowed to such a degree that he or she has no influence over his environment. The more people feel in control of their environment, the lower their level of stress. Stress is greatly alleviated by giving employees an active role in the decision-making process, sharing responsibility, and optimizing the fit between worker needs, abilities, and project demands.

Results are best when the changes—such as improving the work organization in order to avoid overtaxing one department or individual—are made through group process, rather than as a directive from management.

One study of a broad cross-section of workers found that employees often unsuccessfully tried to convince management of better ways to organize task assignments. But because they were consistently ignored, employees tended to give up and do just enough to ensure they received their paycheck at the end of the week. Employees who participate in decision-making and are given more autonomy can become healthier and more productive. A survey of white-collar workers in Sweden reported that those given increased voice in decisions had fewer coronary heart diseases and depression and a 50 percent reduction in absenteeism (International Labor Office, 1993). The conclusion drawn by the 1993 United Nations World Labor Report is that those companies which help employees cope with stress individually and also reengineer the workplace to better suit human aptitudes and aspirations will be the most successful in productivity and in enhancing people's work lives.

Employees, initially happy with their job, often begin to feel uneasy about a situation. If there is no structure set up to hear minor grievances, the unease festers, gradually becoming an unpleasant irritant, perhaps mushrooming into a serious stressor.

> *Cynthia is an employee who was disturbed by ecological waste such as no recycling of inter-office communications and misprints at the Xerox machine. She mentioned it to management, but received no response or encouragement. This unresolved minor dissatisfaction began to color her view of management. As more annoyances accumulated with no avenue of communication, she began to feel insignificant and unappreciated. She ignored her deteriorating morale, but it eventually surfaced as anger and exhaustion.*
>
> *The cause of her stress was not addressed: an organizational structure built around the concept that answers only flow from the top down. Gradually, out of frustration from being unable to effect any change, her enthusiasm for her job dwindled, and she began considering employment elsewhere.*

Management is left with the cost of rehiring and retraining for the vacated position. This example epitomizes what can happen when the organization does not accommodate the need for employees to have some control in their environment. Good business requires abundant, open communication within and across all levels of an organization, with its customers and with its community (California Task Force, 1992).

How I Applied These Principles to the Classroom

Many years ago, at the closing ceremony of a stress management course, I was deeply touched by a gift presented to me by the class. One student played an inspiring melody on the guitar that she had composed, and the others sang in beautiful harmony. Of all the gifts I have received from classes, this one I treasure the most. It taught me an important lesson:

for leadership to be truly successful, there must be room for creative expression and input from the rest of the group. Although I knew my subject well and was benevolent, I was still a dictator. Information and structure for my classes came from the top down. I had all the answers (so I thought!). When I heard the class play and sing together, I realized how much we had lost by my not knowing the skill of one of the students. How much more the class would have benefited if I had known of her ability and incorporated music into the three-month program. In my next class at the University of California I asked if any student could play music. For the whole semester, once a week, different students played music—guitar, flute, recorder, cello, shakuhachi, harp—while I guided the class through deep relaxation and visualization. It was a wonderful success, far beyond the music itself.

I now make a conscious effort in every course I teach to draw on the innate talents and previous training of the students. I have never been disappointed. I still essentially lead the classes, but the structure is flexible, and communication flows in two directions. There is much more participation by the students, and I often delegate projects to an individual or small group. The traditional lecture approach—with the students taking notes and then spitting back "the truth according to Valerie"—has been replaced with brainstorming and input from the students. This has greatly increased the success of the classes. The art of effective teaching lies not only in leading the class, but also in reflecting and magnifying the talents of the group.

I have found this approach successful also in counseling. Although part of my role is advisory and educational in nature, real change in clients comes when I empower them to reach their own highest potential.

Empowering the Employee Rewards Everyone

This team approach is also effective in the business world. The best way to attain long-term financial goals is not through direct, rigid control by management. Pushing the employee to get the most out of him does not work. Attitudes that do not encourage a give-and-take relationship, and assume that leadership knows best, fail to capitalize on the potential contribution of each employee. If company values reflect trust and positive expectation, then the highest qualities and skills of the employees blossom. Shoddy workmanship, mediocrity, and sabotage are expressions of anger or defeat. People need to have a voice in the workplace. They need to be acknowledged and appreciated for their input. Loyalty, hard work, and creativity evolve out of shared responsibility, flexibility, and open communication. This is illustrated by the surprising breakthroughs in creativity that occur when people are given responsibility for their actions. Over and over again, people who never gave any indication of creativity will come through in amazing ways when they are given the opportunity (Society for the Advancement of the Human Spirit, 1992).

Genuine leadership is of only one type: supportive. It leads people: it doesn't drive them. It involves them: it doesn't coerce them. It never loses sight of the most important principle governing any project involving human beings: namely, that people are more important than things (Walters, 1992).

Enhancing Employee Self-Esteem

The central guiding concept for management to promote wellness at work is to promote the self-esteem of all employees. Fundamental to the creation of a healthy atmosphere is the assurance of all workers of their importance. This means soliciting and encouraging their ideas, especially pertaining to their own jobs (Cohen, 1989).

> *Sarah, one of the 15 to 18 million clerical workers and secretaries in the United States, came into counseling complaining about her low pay, repetitive work, and low level of physical activity. She was depressed because she was unchallenged at her work and bored. She could see no possibility of career advancement and was not asked to participate in any organizational decisions. "I'm not valued as a total person. No one asks for my suggestions. They don't involve me in the organization. I'm treated as a commodity, not an intelligent human being. Nobody gives a damn about me."*

Sarah represents untapped potential in her company. People perform best when they are encouraged, included, listened to, and valued. People are the very life force of your company. That life force is most vital when acknowledged and esteemed. Employee potential is maximized in an atmosphere that is supportive. The natural results are improved morale, reduced absenteeism, and increased efficiency.

Cooperation and consideration from the top down is contagious. Esteem can be shown in small ways as well as large. The simple act of supervisors or managers answering phones during lunch to allow clericals to take lunch breaks with friends rather than eat alone is a small example. The camaraderie creates a feeling of belonging, increases self-worth, and makes the job more enjoyable (Cohen, 1989).

When a person comes in for counseling due to anxiety or depression, one of the primary concerns is whether or not the client has a personal support system. Adverse working conditions can be offset by the support of coworkers or supervisors. Opportunities for socializing and sharing task assignments help employees establish personal connections with fellow workers. A support system of friends at work moderates adverse work conditions and buffers the effects of depression and job dissatisfaction.

In a survey conducted by the California Department of Mental Health, self-esteem was significantly related to physical and emotional well-being. Its report concluded that workplace environments and training programs which nurture self-esteem result in higher productivity and markedly reduced absenteeism (California Task Force, 1992).

The bipartisan California Task Force to Promote Self-Esteem and Personal and Social Responsibility spent three years searching out root causes of our social problems and ways to prevent them. From its public hearings it became evident to the Task Force that corporate policy and procedure have a crucial impact on self-worth, dignity, and responsibility felt by employees. After extensive testimony and months of deliberation, the Task Force defined self-esteem as "appreciating my own worth and importance and having the character to be accountable for myself and to act responsibly toward others" (California Task Force, 1992).

"Appreciating my own worth and importance" means recognizing and respecting one's own innate worth as a unique human being. It means accepting ourselves, acknowledging our strengths and weaknesses. It is only in accepting ourselves that we can move forward and change. In owning our past and forgiving others and/or ourselves, we can release pain and be more fully in the present and future, setting reasonable goals and expectations for ourselves, trusting ourselves, and appreciating our creativity. Appreciating our worth also means validating our feelings by risking expression of them to others.

"Having the character to be accountable for myself" means integrity in my actions—that is, accepting responsibility for my actions and the consequences of my behavior. It means taking risks based on faith in my judgment. It means listening to others, but taking responsibility for my choices, not blaming others for influencing my final decisions and actions.

"To act responsibly towards others" is being trustworthy and reliable. Others come to recognize your accountability, that you will follow through on what you commit to, and will assume responsibility for the results.

Virginia Satir, family therapist and renowned author and lecturer on self-esteem, stated that self-esteem can flourish only in an atmosphere where individual differences are appreciated, mistakes are tolerated, communication is open, and rules are flexible (California Task Force, 1992). Workplace policy and procedure based on these principles promote employee self-esteem, result in higher productivity, and reduce absenteeism. Enlightened management shows that it values its employees (as well as suppliers and customers) through equitable treatment and flexible rules. This promotes mutual respect and improved morale.

As employees come to value themselves, their self-esteem leads them to appreciate and value the unique worth of others, giving them respect, acceptance, and support. They are more likely to cooperate and negotiate. They are more likely to accept emotional expression from others, forgive others, and appreciate them. In short, esteem leads to a superior working environment and a superior business.

A Prescription for Change

Tom Peters, business philosopher and theorist, calls the business community to action in his book, *Thriving in Chaos*. His prescription calls for management enhancement of employee self-esteem. Peters questions the efficacy of demeaning and humiliating employees and then expecting them to care about product quality. Peters' prescription includes the following actions:

1. Involve everyone in everything.

2. Use self-managing teams.

3. Listen to, celebrate, and recognize the individual.

4. Spend considerable time recruiting.

5. Provide in-depth training.

6. Provide incentive pay for everyone.

7. Provide employment guarantees.

8. Simplify and reduce structure.

9. Reconceive the middle manager's role.

10. Eliminate bureaucratic rules and humiliating conditions (Peters, 1987).

Words, deeds, and policies that harm, coerce, control, or break the spirit destroy dignity and hope (Peters, 1987). Meeting both the economic and non-economic needs of the worker in an esteeming manner enriches the life of both the worker and the company. Employees need appreciation not only for their productivity, but for who they are as individuals. Once management accepts this philosophy, the details of implementation appropriate to a particular company will unfold naturally.

Conclusion

Management can effectively contribute to employee wellness at work. Establishing an EAP or Wellness Program, implementing structural changes, and respecting employees curtails employee stress and has a positive impact on the corporation. Reducing employee job stress promotes a healthy company on all levels.

Epilogue

You cannot perceive beauty but with a serene mind.

—Henry David Thoreau

Like a flower seeking the sun, we long to identify with the possibility of who we can be. Our shadow self pushes us to change for the better. Underlying all that we do is our work towards self-fulfillment and the diminishing of that which is not our true or highest self. How we relate to this life work is our biggest challenge and is what gives meaning to our lives.

Sometimes daily stress nips our desire for self-betterment in the bud. But if we can remember the longer rhythm of our lives, if we can get appropriate help when needed, and if we can learn to be patient with ourselves, each of us can overcome these obstacles and blossom into the person we desire to be.

I hope *Wellness at Work* helps you facilitate this growth process by helping you manage your stress. Come back to it. Review it. Incorporate the techniques into your life and into your job. Use it as a reference to improve your life in a way that makes you feel good about yourself. Stress management at home and at work is a necessary rung in the ladder of personal growth and full expression. When stress is the spice of life that motivates you, rather than a poison that overwhelms you, it empowers you to be who you want to be and to enjoy your work, your relationships, and yourself.

Appendix A

Caffeine Chart

The following chart was presented at the Sleep, Diet, and the Brain Workshop in Sacramento, California, May 1994 (Waterhouse, 1994), as a guideline for managing stress:

150 - 500 milligrams (mg.) of caffeine contributes to anxiety;
above 500 mg. of caffeine produces anxiety.

Coffee	*Caffeine in milligrams (mg.)*
Espresso	350
Drip - 10 oz. cup	360
Percolate - 10 oz. cup	220
Instant - 10 oz. cup	132
Decaffeinated - 10 oz.	4
Tea	
1-min. brew, bag - 5 oz.	28
5-min. brew, bag - 5 oz.	46
Loose tea 5 min. brew	4
Canned iced tea - 12 oz.	29

Cocoa and Chocolate	*Caffeine in milligrams (mg.)*
Cocoa - 5 oz.	13
Chocolate milk - 10 oz.	2
Choc. fudge topping - 2 tbls.	5
Milk chocolate - 1 oz.	6
Baking chocolate - 1 oz.	35
Dark chocolate - 1 oz.	20

Soft Drinks - 12 oz. Can	
Diet Mr. Pibb	52
Mountain Dew	52
Tab	44
Shasta Cola, Sunkist Orange	42
Dr. Pepper	38
Diet Dr. Pepper	37
Pepsi Cola	37
Royal Crown Cola	36
Diet Rite Cola	34
Diet Pepsi	34
Coca-Cola	34
Mr. Pibb	33
Cragmont Cola	Trace
7-Up, Diet 7-Up	0
Diet Sunkist Orange	0
Patio Orange	0
Fanta Orange	0
Fresca	0
Hires Root Beer	0

Non-Prescription Drugs; Stimulants (per tablet)	Caffeine in milligrams (mg.)
Caffedrine capsules	200
No-Doz tablets	200
Vivarin tablets	200
Pain Relievers (per tablet)	
Anacin	32
Exedrin	64
Midol	32
Plain aspirin	0
Vanquish	33
Diuretics (per tablet)	
Agua-ban	100
Pre-Mens Forte	100
Permathene H20 off	200
Cold Remedies	
Dristan (per tablet)	32
Coryban-D (std. dose)	30
Triaminic (std. dose)	30
Duradyne - Forte	30
Weight-Control Aids (daily dose)	
Dexatrim	200
Dietac	200
Prolamine	280
Appedrine	100

Appendix B

The Facts About Smoking

Smoking *is* bad for your health! One out of every six deaths in the United States is related to tobacco (Northrup, 1994). According to the American Cancer Society and the federal Centers for Disease Control and Prevention, the act of smoking raises your blood pressure and pulse rate, and constricts flow of blood to the hands and feet. It raises the level of carbon monoxide in the body and reduces oxygen levels. Deadly diseases are caused by these metabolic changes. If you lead a stressful, sedentary life, and have a genetic history of a systemic illness, smoking is an additional extremely important risk factor.

What happens when you quit smoking? According to extensive research, the following metabolic processes are normalized.

Consider these American Cancer Society statistics (Jacob, 1993):

Within 20 minutes of your last cigarette, your pulse rate and blood pressure, elevated by nicotine, returns to normal. Circulation in your hands and feet improve.

Within eight hours the oxygen level in your bloodstream will rise and carbon monoxide will drop to its normal level.

Within 24 hours your chance of a heart attack decreases.

Within three days you will breathe easier. Your smoker's breath disappears, and your nerve endings start regrowing. Your ability to taste and smell improves within several days.

Within several months circulation improves, and lung function increases up to 30 percent. Sinus congestion and shortness of breath decrease. Walking becomes easier and you will feel more energetic.

Within one year excess risk of coronary heart disease is half that of when you were smoking.

Within two years your risk of heart attack drops to near normal.

Within five years the lung cancer death rate for someone who was smoking one pack a day decreases by almost 50 percent. Risk of a stroke is reduced to that of a non smoker.

5 to 15 years after quitting risk of cancer of the mouth, throat, and esophagus is half that of a smoker's.

Within 10 years your lung cancer death rate is similar to that of the non smoker. Precancerous cells are replaced. Risk of cancer of the mouth, throat, esophagus, bladder, kidney, and pancreas decreases.

Within 15 years your risk of coronary heart disease is that of a non smoker's.

Appendix C

Calcium Rich Foods

The following chart is adapted from information found in *Women's Bodies, Women's Wisdom* (Northrup, 1994) and *Let's Eat Right to Keep Fit* (Davis, 1970).

Green Leafy Vegetables (1 cup, cooked)	*Calcium—in milligrams (mg.)*
Artichoke, one large globe	50
Bok choy	200
Beet greens	165
Chard	155
Collard greens	300
Spinach	278

Other Vegetables (1 cup, cooked)	
Broccoli	150
Carrots, diced	38
Celery, 1 large stalk	54
Parsnips	88

Sea Vegetables	*Calcium—in milligrams (mg.)*
(available in health food stores)	
Hijiki, 1 cup, cooked	610
Wakame, 1 cup, cooked	520
Kombu (kelp) 1 cup, cooked	305

Fruit

Orange, 1 medium	50
Dates, 1 cup	105
Fig, 1 large, dried	40
Green olives, 5 large, bottled	35

Beans and Legumes

Tofu, firm - 4 oz.	80-150
Black beans - 1 cup, cooked	135
Green snap beans - 1 cup, cooked	45
Kidney beans - 1 cup, canned	74
Pinto beans- 1 cup, cooked	128
Corn tortillas - 2	120

Nuts and Seeds

Almonds - 1 cup	300
Sesame seeds, ground for absorption - 3 tbls.	300
Sunflower seeds, hulled - 1 cup	174

Other Sources

Eggs, 2	54
Salmon, canned - 3 oz.	160
Sardines, canned - 3oz.	367
Shrimp, steamed - 3 oz.	98
Blackstrap molasses - 1 tbs.	137

Dairy	*Calcium—in milligrams (mg.)*
Milk - 1 cup	
Skim	300
Whole	288
Cheese, American, Swiss, cheddar - 1oz.	200
Ice milk - 1 cup	204
Nonfat yogurt - 1 cup	294
Cottage cheese, low fat - 1 cup	150

References

Adler, T. 1993a. "Psychologists in the Trenches Report on Layoffs." *The APA Monitor* 24:8 (August).

Adler, T. 1993b. "Layoffs Just Part of Downsizing Formula." *The APA Monitor* 24:8 (August).

Airola, P. 1981. *How to Get Well*. Phoenix, AZ: Health Plus Publishers.

The Almacan (August 1989), "McDonnell Douglas Corporation's EAP Produces Hard Data."

American College of Sports Medicine. 1993. "Experts Release New Recommendations to Fight America's Epidemic of Physical Inactivity." *News Release* (29 July).

Bailey, C. 1991. *The New Fit or Fat*. Boston: Houghton Mifflin.

Benson, H. 1976. *The Relaxation Response*. New York: Avon Books.

Berkeley Health Letters Associates. 1990. *Wellness Made Easy*. Berkeley, CA: University of California.

Blanchard, K. 1982. *The One-Minute Manager*. New York: William Morrow.

Boga, S. 1993. *Adventure Athletes: Runners and Walkers*. Harrisburg, PA: Stackpole Books.

Borysenko, J. 1987. *Minding the Body, Mending the Mind*. Reading, MA: Addison-Wesley.

Bradshaw, John. 1990. *Homecoming*. New York: Bantam Books.

Braillier, L. 1982. "Transition and Transformation: Successfully Managing Stress." *National Nursing Review*.

Burns, D. 1980. *Feeling Good: The New Mood Therapy.* New York: New American Library.

California Department of Mental Health. 1981. *Friends Can Be Good Medicine.* San Francisco: Pacificon Productions.

California Task Force to Promote Self-Esteem and Personal and Social Responsibility. 1992. *Toward a State of Esteem.* Sacramento, CA: California State Department of Education.

California Workers' Compensation Institute. 1990. "Mental Stress Claims in California Workers' Compensation—Incidents, Costs, and Trends." *California Workers' Compensation Institute Research Notes* (June).

Cannon, J. 1992. *What's Right With Your Life? Wellness Appraisal.* Chicago: Inward Bound Ventures.

Castro, J. 1993. "What Price Mental Health?" *Time* Magazine (31 May).

Cohen, B.G.F. 1989. "Organizational Factors Affecting Stress in the Clerical Worker." In *Human Aspects of Office Automation* edited by B.G.F. Cohen. Amsterdam, Netherlands: Elsevier Science Publishers (Obtainable through the National Institute of Mental Health, Washington, D.C.).

Consumer Reports (February 1993). "Can Your Body Heal Your Mind?"

Cooper, H., MD. 1978. *The Aerobics Way.* New York: Bantam Books.

Cornell, J. 1987. *Listening to Nature.* Nevada City, CA: Dawn Publications.

Cousins, N. 1990. "A Nation of Hypochondriacs." *Time* Magazine (18 June).

Davis, A. 1970. *Let's Eat Right to Keep Fit.* New York: Harcourt, Brace Jovanovich.

Davis, M., E.R. Eshelman, and M. McKay. 1988. *The Relaxation & Stress Reduction Workbook,* 3rd ed. Oakland, CA: New Harbinger Publications.

DSM-IV (Diagnostical Statistical Manual of Mental Disorders, 4th ed.). 1994. Washington, D.C.: American Psychiatric Association.

Dunkin, A., ed. 1993. "Meditation, The New Balm for Corporate Stress." *Business Week* (10 May).

Eisenberg, D.M. et al. 1993. "Unconventional Medicine in the United States: Prevalence, Costs, and Patterns of Use." *New England Journal of Medicine* (28 January).

Fahrion, S.L., and P.A. Norris. 1990. "Self-Regulation of Anxiety." *Bulletin of the Menninger Clinic* 54.

Gibbs, N. 1989. "How America Has Run Out of Time." *Time* Magazine (24 April).

Green, J. 1988. *Biofeedback Training: A Client Information Paper.* Wheat Ridge, CO: Association for Applied Psychophysiology and Biofeedback.

International Labor Office. 1993. "Stress at Work." In *United Nations World Labor Report*. Geneva: International Labor Office.

Jacob, B. 1993. "Reaping Rewards from the Great American Smokeout." *Vitality* 7:11 (November).

Jacobson, E. 1938. *Progressive Relaxation*. Chicago: University of Chicago Press.

Jones, T. 1980. *Employee Assistance Programs in Industry*. Phoenix, AZ: Do It Now Foundation.

Kaufman, B.N. 1991. *Happiness Is a Choice*. New York: Ballantine Books.

King, A.G. 1995. "Employee Assistance Program on the Rise." *USA Today* (1 May).

Klarreich, S.H. 1990. *Work Without Stress*. New York: Brunner/Mazel Publishers.

Korn, P. 1994. "Health Risks at 20, 30, 40, 50, 60, 70+." *Self* (September).

Kriyananda, S. 1991. *Yoga Postures for Higher Awareness*. Nevada City, CA: Crystal Clarity Publishers.

Lowlier, J. 1993. "Meditation 'takes the edge off' at Work." *USA Today* (18 June).

Marx, J.L. 1990. In "Prevention of Work-Related Psychological Disorders," by S.L. Sauter, et al. *American Psychologist* 45:10 (October).

McKay, M. and P. Fanning. 1992. *Prisoners of Belief*. Oakland, CA: New Harbinger Publications.

Menninger Clinic, Center for Applied Psychophysiology. n.d. "Breathing and the Stress Response" (handout). Topeka, KS: The Menninger Clinic, Center for Applied Psychophysiology.

New Ways to Work Publications. 1993. "New Ways to Work." San Francisco: New Ways to Work Publications.

Norris, P.A. 1986. "Biofeedback, Voluntary Control, and Human Potential." *Biofeedback and Self-Regulation* 11:1.

Norris, P.A. 1989a. "Clinical Psychoneuroimmunology: Strategies for Self-Regulation of Immune System Responding." In *Biofeedback Principles and Practice for Clinicians*, edited by J.V. Basmajian. Baltimore, MD: Williams and Wilkins.

Norris, P.A. 1989b. "Current Conceptual Trends in Biofeedback and Self-Regulation." In *Eastern and Western Approaches to Healing*, edited by A. Sheikh. New York: John Wiley and Sons.

Norris, P.A. 1989c. "Healing: What We Can Learn From Children." In *Healers on Healing*, edited by R. Carlson and B. Shield. Los Angeles: Jeremy P. Tarcher.

Norris, P.A., and S.L. Fahrion. 1993. "Autogenic Biofeedback in Psychophysiological Therapy and Stress Management." In *Principles and Practices of Stress Management*, P.M. Lehrer and R.L. Woolfolk. New York: The Guilford Press.

Northrup, C. 1994. *Women's Bodies, Women's Wisdom.* New York: Bantam Books.

The Office of Alternative Medicine. 1992. *Functional Description Paper.* Bethesda, MD: The Office of Alternative Medicine.

O'Hara, V. 1990. *The Fitness Option.* Nevada City, CA: Dawn Publications.

Painton, P. 1993. "Couch Potatoes Arise." *Time* Magazine (9 August).

Paul, S.C. 1991. *Illuminations.* San Francisco: Harper and Row.

Pawlak, L. 1993. *Tomorrow's Woman.* Cathedral City, CA: Laura Pawlak.

Pelletier, K.R. 1982. *Mind As Healer, Mind As Slayer.* New York: Dell Publishing.

Peters, T. 1987. *Thriving in Chaos.* New York: Alfred A Knopf.

Phillips, G. 1988. *Think Light!* San Diego, CA: Speaking of Fitness, Inc.

President's Council on Physical Fitness and Sports. 1993a. *Adult Fitness Fact Sheet.* Washington, D.C.: President's Council on Physical Fitness and Sports.

President's Council on Physical Fitness and Sports. 1993b. "Heart Center Supports 'Commit to Get Fit.'" *Newsletter* (Spring).

President's Council on Physical Fitness and Sports. 1993c. *Employee Fitness Fact Sheet.* Washington, D.C.: President's Council on Physical Fitness and Sports.

President's Council on Physical Fitness and Sports. 1993d. *One Step at a Time.* Washington, D.C.: President's Council on Physical Fitness and Sports.

Preston, J. 1993. *Growing Beyond Emotional Pain.* San Luis Obispo, CA: Impact Publishers.

Regier, D.A., MD; W.E. Narrow, MD, MPH; D.S. Rae, MA; R.W. Manderscheid, PhD; D.Z. Locke, MSPH; and F.K. Goodwin, MD. 1993. "The de facto U.S. Mental and Addictive Disorders Service System." *Archives of General Psychiatry* 50 (February).

Regier, D.A., MD; J.K. Meyer, M. Kramer, L.N. Robins, D.G. Blazer, R.L. Hough, W.W. Eaton, and B.Z. Locke. 1984. "The NIMH Epidemiologic Catchment Area (ECA) Program: Historical Context, Major Objectives, and Study Population Characteristics." *Archives of General Psychiatry* 41:10 (October).

Sauter, S.L., L.R. Murphy, and J.J. Hurrell, Jr. 1990. "Prevention of Work-Related Psychological Disorders." *American Psychologist* 45:10 (October)

Society for the Advancement of the Human Spirit. 1992. *Society for the Advancement of the Human Spirit Proposal and Action Plan.* Newport Beach, CA: Society for the Advancement of the Human Spirit.

Taub, E., MD. 1988. *Prescription for Life.* Sausalito, CA: American Wellness Association.

Trafford, A.P. 1993. *The Heroic Path.* Carson, CA: Hay House, Inc.

Tubesing, N.L. and D.A. Tubesing. 1990. *Structured Exercises in Stress Management,* vol. 1. Duluth, MN: Whole Person Press.

U.S. Department of Labor; Bureau of Labor Statistics. 1993. "Employment and Earnings Characteristics of Families: Second Quarter, 1993." *News* (20 July).

U.S. Department of Health and Human Services. 1990. *Drug Abuse Curriculum for Employee Assistance Program Professionals.* Rockville, MD: U.S. Department of Health and Human Services.

Walker, C.K. 1991. "Stressed to Kill." *Business and Health* (September).

Wallace, J. 1992. "Reduce Job Stress Before It Reduces You." *Safety and Health* (November).

Walters, J.D. 1989. *Secrets of Overcoming Harmful Emotions.* Nevada City, CA: Crystal Clarity Publishers.

Waterhouse, D.L. 1994. "Caffeine Chart." In paper presented at the Sleep, Diet, and the Brain Workshop, May 1994, at Sacramento, CA.

Witmer, J.M., and T.J. Sweeney. 1992. "A Holistic Model for Wellness and Prevention Over the Life Span." *Journal of Counseling and Development* 71:2 (November/December).

Zeff, T. 1981. *The Psychological and Physiological Effects of Meditation and the Physical Isolation Tank Experience on the Type A Behavior Pattern.* (dissertation) San Francisco: California Institute of Integral Studies.